ENDORSEMENT

"Fifty years ago, the American Heart Association began a series of recommendations for changes in the American diet to help in the prevention of heart disease. The central feature of those recommendations was the reduction of animal fat. The most dramatic and effective change in that effort is simply to consume only foods from vegetable sources. Although that was not the specific recommendation of the AHA, the assumption of a vegetarian eating pattern was accepted as a reasonable choice to achieve reduced heart attacks and strokes. *The 95% Vegan Diet* provides a clearly stated rationale that is in agreement with our national guidelines for dietary change and provides a number of practical and realistic choices that can help transition from a diet high in meat and dairy products to one that is predominately from vegetable sources. There is also the recognition that being religiously perfect in eating only fruits and vegetables is not necessary to be successful in gaining a lower blood cholesterol and possibly a lower blood pressure as well as a lower body weight. These benefits can result from gradual changes to one with much less fat from animal sources. The importance of these considerations is the recognition that preventable vascular disease is now the number one cause of death in the entire world."

—W. Virgil Brown, M.D.,
Professor of Medicine Emeritus,
Emory University School of Medicine,
and past president of The American Heart Association
and the National Board of Clinical Lipidology

"The 95% Vegan Diet provides a template for those who want to experience the therapeutic benefits of a vegan diet, without completely eliminating animal products. It is beautifully written and wonderfully interactive. The author draws from her unique experience as both a dietitian and a clinical pharmaceutical researcher to provide practical insights that will make your journey to health a pleasure."

—Brenda Davis, RD,
Author of *Becoming Vegetarian,*
Becoming Vegan, and *Becoming Raw*

"If you're someone who's considered a plant-based diet but doesn't quite feel up to a '30 day vegan challenge,' try Jamie's positively friendly, non-judgmental, easy approach. Jamie holds your hand as she walks you through an overview of vegan nutrition, cooking, and health, helping you ease into a new way of eating at your pace. She seems to understand the concerns of the reader, and addresses them with care and thoroughness."

—Miyoko Schinner,
Author of *Artisan Vegan Cheese, Japanese Cooking:*
Contemporary & Traditional
[Simple, Delicious, and Vegan], and *The New Now and Zen*
Epicure: Gourmet Vegan Recipes for the Enlightened Palate

"If you're not sure how or why to go vegan, *The 95% Vegan Diet* breaks down the medical facts into bite-sized pieces. Your doctor may be telling you to cut out meat and this book is a how-to manual to making a diet transition. From the whys of being vegan to setting up your kitchen all the way to the easy to make recipes in the appendix you'll find all the information you need to make your diet change easier and more maintainable.

—Kathy Hester,
author of *The Vegan Slow Cooker* and
The Great Vegan Bean Book

THE 95% VEGAN DIET

-DIET-

THE 95% VEGAN DIET

-DIET-

AN INSIDER'S GUIDE TO TAKING
CONTROL OF YOUR DIET AND HEALTH
WITHOUT HAVING TO BE PERFECT

JAMIE NOLL, PHARM. D., LD, CDE AND CAITLIN E. HERNDON, JD

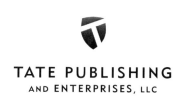

TATE PUBLISHING
AND ENTERPRISES, LLC

Published by Tate Publishing & Enterprises, LLC
127 E. Trade Center Terrace | Mustang, Oklahoma 73064 USA
1.888.361.9473 | www.tatepublishing.com

Tate Publishing is committed to excellence in the publishing industry. The company reflects the philosophy established by the founders, based on Psalm 68:11,
"The Lord gave the word and great was the company of those who published it."

Book design copyright © 2013 by Tate Publishing, LLC. All rights reserved.
Cover design by Ronnel Luspoc
Interior design by Caypeeline Casas

Published in the United States of America
ISBN: 978-1-62563-816-8
1. Health & Fitness / Diet & Nutrition / General
2. Cooking / Vegetarian & Vegan
13.07.29

DEDICATION

· ·

We dedicate this book in loving memory to our parents and grandparents, *James H. and Doris G. Noll.*

Your loving wisdom and visionary commitment to change the face of things, to create a ripple effect for the generations to come, will never be forgotten.

ACKNOWLEDGMENTS

We have been divinely blessed to have so many wonderful people in our lives who share our passion for dispersing factual knowledge to help people and improve their journey in life; it is impossible to mention all of them. For those we do not mention here, we hope you will forgive us and know we meant no disrespect. We hold all of our loving family and friends very dear.

We would first like to acknowledge Tate Publishing and Enterprises for believing in this book and in us. From our first encounter with Noel Thrasher, acquisitions editor, to our talented project manager, Rachael Sweeden, to layout, cover design and final stages of editing with Kyle Crawford and Chris Webb, it has been our joy to work with this publishing company.

Throughout the writing of this book, several of our dear friends and colleagues have provided assistance, which significantly improved the book's contents and helped build the *95% Vegan* concept. To that end, we would like to thank Lisa Kerr, both for her expertise as a statistician and for her unyielding friendship; Marcy Saucedo for her design of the original logo and for relentlessly sharing her artistic talent, love, and belief; and Dale Holderfield, Pharm. D., for his clinical review and consistent teaching, mentoring, and friendship. For his critical eye and sharing his expertise in food and drug law, we thank Christopher Lee Hagenbush, JD, adjunct professor of food and drug law at Georgia State University College of Law.

There are always those people who have affected your life tremendously along the way and who provided the opportunity to become the person you are and to possess the skills necessary to create the work you have. In this light, we thank Carolyn D. Berdanier, PhD, professor of nutrition emerita at the University of Georgia; the faculty at Georgia State University College of Law; and the faculty at the University of Georgia College of Pharmacy. We also thank Mary Maloy for providing early career opportunities and then undying friendship for over twenty years. We thank Doug Muchmore, MD, for his true grit, mentoring, and support.

Other people along our journey who helped make this book a reality include Alan Garber, JD, for his unyielding ethics, legal expertise, and consistent support, and Marc Lubatkin, JD, for enabling us to soar to new heights.

We also thank our cousin, Lauren Noll, PhD, for her pure love and devotion, as well as for sharing her vast intelligence and insight to human behavior. We thank Alan Lampe for the many years he has mentored us and been our friend, as well as for sharing his critical eye in finalizing this book.

In the final stages of editing, Rachel Ashe, JD, Lauren Pendley, JD, and Kelly Wright, MPA, provided kind words and valuable feedback for which we are grateful.

We could not have done it without all of those mentioned. Most of all, we could not have done it without our creator and Lord, for *through Him, all things are possible.*

CONTENTS

· ·

PART 2:
First Things First

PART 3:
LET'S DIVE IN!

PART 4:
STRATEGIES FOR SPECIFIC MEDICAL ISSUES

PART 5:
BECOME YOUR OWN SCIENTIST

INTRODUCTION

For whatever reasons you are thinking of going vegan, you are on the right track! There are many examples throughout the world that have provided strong evidence to support the concept that it is the healthiest diet on the planet. People who eat mostly plant-based foods tend to weigh less, and have lower rates of heart disease, diabetes, and some forms of cancer, such as breast, colorectal, and prostate cancers.

But as you think through it, you wonder how you could maintain such a strict regimen over the long haul. How will you survive family gatherings? What about when you travel and are at the mercy of what is available at the destination? Before you give up on the idea, let's examine some realities, and please allow my daughter Caitlin and I to offer another option: to go 95% vegan!

The China Study[1] was a very strong scientific work supporting plant-based nutrition. Drs. T. Colin Campbell and Thomas M. Campbell II provided the world a significant gift with their publication. They did more than present one or two scientific studies; they connected the dots of scientific evidence spanning decades in a means that has the potential to change the downward spiral of our health in the westernized culture. Based on the largest epidemiological study ever conducted, *The China Study* sent a strong signal that a plant-based diet is the healthiest diet in the world. Those groups who consumed a mostly plant-based diet had far lower incidences of the chronic diseases we who live in a westernized culture experience: cardiovascular disease, type 2 diabetes, and certain types of cancer thought to be diet-related.

At the same time, miraculous results in a relatively small group of very sick heart-diseased patients (most had no other hope as they were not candidates for surgery) studied over years by Caldwell B. Esselstyn Jr., MD, and published in his book *Prevent and Reverse Heart Disease*[2] demonstrated that a severely restrictive plant-based diet with zero added fat can prevent and reverse heart disease. To see the proof of reversal of diseased blood vessels on the angiograms is amazing! Dr. Esselstyn has certainly provided the world with powerful evidence of using food as medicine. In fact, the vegan diet is the only therapy now proven to reverse heart disease; no drug has been demonstrated to do what the vegan diet can do.

The highest praise should be given to Dr. Esselstyn for his work, his caring, and his tenacity, for he proved to the world what could be accomplished in an ideal environment. However, due to lack of funding, Dr. Esselstyn was unable to study other groups of patients at the same time to compare the all-or-none approach to one or more less stringent approaches.

Had it been possible, it would have been helpful in Dr. Esselstyn's study to have had two or three other groups with progressively increasing fat intake within the plant-based regimen as well as different percent of intake from calories from meat and dairy sources in order to determine the level that people could get away with and still achieve the same results as the more extreme group. For example, Dr. Esselstyn's study group had 0 percent added fat in their diets. They had no nuts, olives, avocados, or other natural foods known to be high in fat. But how do we know that adding 10 percent calories as fat, or 20 or 30 percent added would not have produced significant, if not the same results as 0 percent? The fact is, we don't know because it was not studied at the same time the 0 percent group was studied. The same holds true for meat consumption; we don't know just how vegan the patients could have been and still reversed their heart disease.

Unfortunately, 25 percent of Dr. Esselstyn's patients dropped out the first year because they could not comply with the extreme regimen. It is good that they did drop out so as not to confound the results of the study. However, we can also take away the fact that 25 percent of the sickest cardiac patients with no other hope of living would not comply with such a strict regimen. The 75 percent of remaining patients in his study were seen in the clinic by Dr. Esselstyn every two weeks and had other support, including having quarterly visits to Dr. Esselstyn's home for food and group support. In addition, Dr. Esselstyn had a "my way or the highway" approach—if a patient wanted to fall off the wagon, he or she would be shown to the door. This was necessary, for as we shall see, it is extremely difficult to study nutrition in humans. There are many other variables that could have affected the study results, so strict controls needed to have been in place.

But where else on planet Earth could one find the level of support and consistent reprimands given in Dr. Esselstyn's study? In my experience, that type of care is only seen within the confines of the clinical research world where the studied factor must be isolated by controlling all other factors. In other words, it is unlikely to find that level of support unless one is part of a clinical trial.

What about the average patient who is not currently at death's door, having had multiple heart attacks or strokes and given little time to live? Consider the real world budgets of time and money. How likely would that person be successful with Dr. Esselstyn's approach? Probably not very likely, even if that person knew the dangling carrot, the reward, is the prevention and reversal of heart disease. Consider how many smokers know the risks of smoking yet continue to puff away day in and day out. It is unfortunate, but true: we tend to live for the pleasures of today, and we really hate to inconvenience ourselves.

If you haven't read *The China Study* and *Prevent and Reverse Heart Disease*, I highly recommend that you do. I would also recommend if you don't have the time to read these books to at least watch *Forks Over Knives*[3], a documentary that brilliantly brings together Drs. Campbell's and Esselstyn's work. These works provide a solid basis for you to move forward nutritionally, from credible, scientific sources. While I will provide a brief discussion of some of the evidence that points toward supporting these works in Part 1, the focus of this book is to help you assess your own health and nutritional status and implement what we now know is the healthiest diet on the planet: a low fat, plant-based vegan diet. This diet, especially if combined with any needed weight loss, will make you as cancer-, heart disease-, and diabetes-proof as you can possibly be, and, based on the results from the *Diabetes Prevention Program* study and *Preventing and Reversing Heart Disease*, is more effective prevention than any medicine known to man.

Most of us have two goals. One is that we want to lose weight. The other is that we want to avoid having diseases that are thought to be associated with our unhealthy, westernized diet. These goals are not mutually exclusive. Since both our weight and our dietary consumption of meat and fat are strongly associated with type 2 diabetes, cardiovascular disease, and some cancers, it makes sense that we would like to find a way to lose weight while following a plant-based diet.

So what's the problem? In a nutshell, we are back to where we started: we need to find a means to do all of this that is also agreeable with our lifestyle, long-term.

Let's stop and reflect. Have you ever wondered about people who have tried various diets and say things such as, "I used to be on the (fill-in-the-blank) diet"? How about "I tried the (fill-in-the-blank) diet, and it really worked for me." Yet they are still overweight or otherwise reverted back to their old, unhealthy habits. The very fact that they are still struggling should tell them (and you) that the diet itself was not sustainable. Why was it unsustainable? In my experience, there are three general reasons:

1. The diet was too low in calories, so the person constantly felt as if he or she was starving.

2. The diet narrowed food choices to the extent that it did not fit into his or her life and cultural needs.

3. The diet completely cut out certain foods that the person felt he or she could not continue to live without.

In my nearly three decades of practice as a doctor of pharmacy (Pharm. D.), dietitian, and certified diabetes educator, I have counseled thousands of patients. My typical patient encounters last from one to two hours. During that time, I assess the patient's readiness to learn, ability to comprehend scientific principles, literacy skills, food likes and dislikes, and cultural needs. I also get into their heads to better understand their past dietary history and their knowledge and beliefs about food and nutrition. What have they tried before? How did that work? If it worked, why not just try that again? If it didn't work, why didn't it work? How did they feel when it didn't work?

It is my observation that the #1 cause for patients to give up is what I call The Guilt Factor (TGF). They have given up their favorite food, or they have been extremely hungry for days or weeks. In a weak moment, they either eat a food not on the diet list or eat more food than was called for by the diet. The Guilt Factor kicks in. The person is consumed with feelings of inadequacy and guilt. "I am so bad," "I am such a pig," "I'm never going to be thin again," are all statements I have heard uttered by my patients as they recount what happened. They then tell me about the next days, weeks, or months when they binged and ate far more than they ate even before they started the diet in question. They are in a war with themselves, engaging in self-punishing behavior that ultimately places them in a position worse than before they started.

How do we get around these challenges we face? The answer lies in part by facing the reality in which we live and doing the very best we can. Sounds simple, right? If that is all it takes to get your diet to an optimal point so that you get to the weight you want to be, stave off heart attacks, strokes, diabetes, and cancer, then why is it so difficult? There are several reasons, not the least of which is our own expectations of ourselves, and the guilt we place upon ourselves when we slip. Why is it that if we aren't 100% perfect, we give up on ourselves?

"Excellence does not require perfection."

—Henry James

How many of us started out five or ten pounds overweight, then tried to lose weight only to end up being fifteen pounds overweight? How do we become fifty pounds overweight? Is it because we plunged head-on into daily binges without ever looking up and thinking about what we were doing to ourselves? Rarely. Most of us gave sincere effort to one or more weight loss diets. Many of us joined a gym or started some type of exercise program. Yet our weight and the overall rate of obesity continued to climb.

Now let's turn our attention to chronic disease prevention. Did you know that there are scientifically proven facts about preventing some diseases that are well known in the medical community but are not fiercely implemented in the practice of medicine? The best example I can think of is the fact that almost six out of ten cases of type 2 diabetes are preventable through diet and exercise alone. We have known this since the data from the Diabetes Prevention Program (DPP) were published in 2002[4], yet diabetes (90 percent of which is type 2) kills more people every year than breast cancer and AIDs combined![5] What is keeping people from successfully avoiding this cruel disease? There are several potential explanations.

The most obvious explanation is that the scientific world's knowledge about the fact that type 2 diabetes is preventable is not reaching the public through the medical community. Also consider that preventing diseases is not profitable. For example, drug companies don't make money for preventing diseases; they make money by making drugs that treat diseases. Thus, you will not likely see prime-time commercials discussing how to prevent diabetes sponsored by the pharmaceutical industry. Ditto for the fast food industry. So who would sponsor such a campaign, and at what cost?

Another explanation lies in the reality of how our healthcare system works. Chronic diseases such as diabetes are mostly being managed in a busy primary care physician's office. This setting conflicts with the realities of the needs of the patient. Patients who have or are prone to chronic diseases such as type 2 diabetes require more time. They need to be thoroughly educated about how to keep themselves well. But physicians simply do not have the time to spend with these patients. The busy doctor's office works well for patients who are acutely ill, such as having a strep throat. The physician diagnoses the problem, writes a prescription for an antibiotic, and is off to the next patient. In the United States, doctors are essentially compensated by how many patients they see in a day. They rarely make more money if they spend more time with a patient during the office visit. Unfortunately, this often results in suboptimal care for those who need more time with their doctor in order to better understand what they need to do to keep themselves well. The majority of doctors are doing the very best they can, but they also need to support their families.

The reality is that we can prevent devastating diseases such as type 2 diabetes, cardiovascular disease, and some cancers through diet therapy, a plant-based, low fat diet. Such a diet could also help us lose weight. But we still have the challenge of how we can go vegan in a healthy and sustainable way.

I propose we think in a new way. Why should we hold ourselves to the unattainable goal of being perfect? Isn't that what keeps us failing? Think about this: if people could attain 95% vegan status or even just continually move toward that goal, would that improve their risks for developing the chronic diseases attributable to the western diet (heart disease, diabetes, and some cancers)? Absolutely. If people could lose an average of just 7 percent of their body weight, could they possibly prevent getting type 2 diabetes? You bet; that is exactly what happened in the DPP (Diabetes Prevention Program)! The all-or-none mentality, demanding 100 percent compliance can be deadly if you spend more time failing than succeeding. The 95% mentality is reasonable, healthy, and doable for the long haul.

Don't get me wrong; we should all strive to have 100% plant-based diets with zero added fat. It is the highest goal of all. But as I mentioned earlier, real life and The Guilt Factor (TGF) often cause us to fail. As I also mentioned, we still do not know at what point fat restriction and veganism becomes therapeutic. Could we get away with our diets being 25 percent fat and still avoid heart disease and diabetes? Could we add some animal products to our diet (How about 5 percent of total calories, being 95% vegan?) and still successfully avoid the ravages of heart disease? Better yet, if you eat the average American diet containing 40–60 percent fat, an excessive amount of animal and dairy protein as well as sugar, would striving to be 95% vegan on a daily basis and 25 percent or less fat be a significant improvement? Would it help you lose weight? You bet it would!

So there you have it. You do not necessarily have to "be a vegan." You can be 95% vegan, lose weight, and still enjoy your family functions. Isn't that the best of both worlds? That is what this book is all about: teaching you how to be the healthiest you can be without having to be perfect.

"Perfection is not attainable, but if we chase
perfection we can catch excellence."

—Vince Lombardi

We will discuss these concepts in more depth in Part 1 of this book. Also in Part 1, we will address the fact that while we may be successful as individuals, we also need to change the downward spiraling course of our health in this country overall. We must create a ripple effect for future generations. Unless we teach our children proper nutrition, healthy self-control, and respect for their health, the positive influence this book may have will die with this generation. We need to prepare our children and grandchildren by taking the knowledge we have gained and passing it down by word and example. We need to fully integrate the knowledge into our individual lives and collective cultures in order for it to be successfully replicated, generation-to-generation.

Parts 2 and 3 of this book will provide you with details in order to assess your own health as well as prepare yourself, your family, your kitchen, and your budget to become highly successful with your plant-based diet.

We will then take the how-tos and apply them to the strategies we set for your health in Part 4. Weight loss, diabetes, heart disease, chronic kidney disease, celiac disease, and diverticulosis will all be covered. Note that this book is not in any way intended to take the place of your personal physician; it is intended to supplement your overall health knowledge and to show you how to follow a plant-based diet and continue to be successful in preventing or managing these diseases. Along with *The 95% Vegan Diet Workbook*, this book will enable you to have an ongoing conversation with your personal physician regarding your efforts at preventative medicine and management of any chronic diseases you may already have. I strongly encourage you to partner with your doctor to manage your own health.

I have extensive first-hand experience on the inside workings of the pharmaceutical industry, both in the sales/marketing side of the business, as well as on the medical side as a clinical research scientist. In Part 5, we will address the drug and dietary supplement industries such that you can become your own scientist and effectively review the claims you and your family are bombarded with daily. All of the good nutrition in the world would mean very little if you took a "miracle cure" or "ancient herb" that caused your liver or kidneys to fail. Given that these possibilities are real and have been well documented, this is not an alarmist point of view.

As the scientist/clinician, I will walk you through all of the health aspects of the vegan diet, as well as how to evaluate clinical studies. As the lawyer and chief creative kitchen person, Caitlin will discuss food and drug law, as well as share many creative original recipes. She also writes about the vegan food budget and how to have vegan frugal fun throughout all of the seasons of the year. We recommend you read this book from start to finish, rather than jumping from section to section. The reason for this is that there are Homework assignments throughout the book that incrementally build your knowledge so that when you are finished, you should feel very well-prepared to move forward with your health resolutions.

And so, let's compare the journey upon which we are about to embark to a vacation to your favorite destination. You first plan your trip and then arrange your travel by booking a flight or grabbing a map or GPS. You think about what you want to wear daily and to any special events that may be occurring. You do the work; you pack, get on the plane, walk, or take a train, bus, or cab until you finally arrive at the beautiful resort, campground, or cottage. Once there, you enjoy all the fruits of your labor. You may have forgotten to bring a sweater, so you buy one along the way. No matter, it doesn't in any way change the destination or the overall goal of finding relaxation. In other words, the trip itself might not be perfect, but the destination and its rewards remain the same. Likewise, you will first identify your nutritional destination through sound scientific principles. You will think through how you will be most successful daily and on special occasions. You will do the work by preparing food and teaching your family. You will ultimately reap the benefits of being as cancer-proof, heart disease-proof and diabetes-proof as possible. Again, the trip might not be perfect as you may occasionally deviate from your planned diet, but if you continue to move forward, it won't change the "destination"—the overall health outcomes for you or your family.

I hope this introduction has touched your heart, touched a nerve, and challenged your thinking, but, most of all, provided encouragement. I wish you the very best on this journey as you travel to your chosen nutritional destination.

Jamie Noll, Pharm. D., LD, CDE

PART 1:
A Marriage of Science, Society, and Your Realities

MY STORY

I was sitting in a crowded meeting hall at the 70th Scientific Session of the American Diabetes Association in Orlando, Florida. For the last several years, I had been working hard to prove my value as a clinical research scientist on the global diabetes platform at a large pharmaceutical company, but in musing about how much I missed working directly with patients, I decided to attend more presentations related to current trends in patient care outside of drug therapy. My colleagues wondered where I was when I did not show up for any of the typically highly attended drug lectures or the symposia sponsored by competitors. They would have found me in the meetings focused on nutrition, pathology, epidemiology, and public health. I needed to get back to my patients.

The Physicians Committee for Responsible Medicine (PCRM) sponsored one of the lectures I attended on that day. They were presenting the results from a study conducted on GEICO employees, which compared two groups of overweight GEICO employees with or without diabetes. One group consumed a low fat vegan diet, while a control group of employees from a different GEICO office site had no dietary intervention.[1]

The results were astounding. Even though the vegan group ate roughly the same amount of calories as the control group, they lost a significant amount of weight, significantly reduced their waist:hip ratio and significantly lowered their blood pressure. All of these are markers for cardiovascular disease, including heart attack and stroke. Since both of my parents died untimely deaths due to cardiovascular disease, I had a personal stake in understanding any data around its prevention. In addition, my daughter Caitlin was discovered to have insulin resistance when she was only thirteen years of age, putting her at an even greater risk for cardiovascular disease than I am. This risk in my only child increased my attention to all of the data exponentially.

From that lecture, I went to every other lecture involving plant-based diets I could find. The PCRM seemed to have a big presence at that meeting, including a booth on the exhibit floor. As I tried to get my brain wrapped around the concept of cutting all animal products out of our diet, I kept struggling with the concept of not having dairy products in my life. When I was growing up, I was known as the biggest milk drinker in my family. Milk, cheese, yogurt, ice cream, and puddings were the mainstays of my diet. It would be difficult enough giving up those juicy steaks, turkey at Thanksgiving, hot dogs from the street vendors in New York City, and pastrami on rye bread, but milk products? I thought perhaps I would just take my chances with the cardio-vascular risks ahead.

She was like a beacon of light. Brenda Davis, RD, author of *Becoming Vegan*[2] (among other wonderful books on nutrition) was in the PCRM booth, as I happened to go by. We started to chat about the wonderful clinical data being presented around plant-based diets. I lowered my voice and said to her, "Brenda, this is all well and good, but how would someone like me, a dairy queen, ever successfully move to a completely plant-based diet? I could literally eat a pound of cheese a day."

Without missing a beat, she said, "The first thing you need to do is get *The Uncheese Cookbook*[3]." She went on to tell me about the fabulous recipes in the book to substitute for all kinds of cheese and how she had just served a completely vegan meal at a recent party using many of the recipes in the book and how no one guessed that it was not real cheese. That was encouraging.

Brenda then also picked up a copy of *The China Study* [4] and said, "You also need to read this book."

"Okay," I said, now mesmerized by the concept of actually going back to spending more of my time planning my family's nutritional intake. I had been so busy focusing on my career that I had gotten completely off-track.

A couple of days later as I was traveling home, my flight was delayed by several hours. As often happened when I was caught up on my work and stuck in an airport, I found myself on Amazon.com, this time investigating vegan cookbooks. Of course I ordered *The China Study* and *The Uncheese Cookbook*, but I also found several other provocative vegan cookbooks that found their way into my shopping cart. My interest had been significantly heightened with the knowledge that there was so much nutritional and culinary information that had passed under my radar as I chased other priorities. How could I have missed it? I had been a licensed dietitian at that point for over twenty-five years. I had to have thirty hours of continuing education in order to keep my license current every two years. However, since I also had a pharmacist license with the same requirements, I always completed continuing education programs that would cover both licenses at the same time. Those programs could not be strictly nutritional, as it would not satisfy the pharmacist license. Coupled with other priorities, I was a bit out of date on my nutritional knowledge concerning the benefits of a plant-based diet.

Then I read *The China Study*, and my life changed literally overnight. It was as if I had been living in an area that was cold and rainy every day for years, and then suddenly, the sun came out. Flowers bloomed, birds were singing, the air smelled fresh, and the sun shone on my face. The night I finished reading the book, I stayed up all night long just removing every food item that contained animal products from my refrigerator and pantry. By 6:00 a.m., I had four large paper grocery bags full of items I would cut out of my diet.

I became vegan that very day, cold turkey. Being a dietitian armed with several fantastic vegan cookbooks (see Appendix 1 for suggested resources), I found it fairly easy to do. I also discovered that low fat vanilla soymilk was a satisfactory substitute for the gallon of cow's milk I usually consumed every day and a half. Over the next few weeks, I felt hungry, for what seemed like all of the time. No surprise to me; I had been so full, so satiated from the animal protein and saturated fat in my previously unhealthy diet that my new very low fat diet had me feeling hungry. The good news was that I found I was hungry for the fruits and vegetables that were now in my diet. Then it hit me: the reason more of us don't get enough fruits and vegetables in our diets is probably because we simply aren't hungry enough to want them. It is like the child who wants to fill up on macaroni and cheese while completely ignoring the vegetables on his or her plate. Does this sound reasonable to you? It did to me.

The hunger lasted for about three months. That was the hardest part.

About a month into the vegan diet, I realized I had not taken any ibuprofen or glucosamine for about three weeks. That was weird. I had been taking these pills every day for about a year when I started the vegan diet. I thought the aches and pains just signaled middle age. I had been asleep at the wheel for years, evidently, as I did not connect my huge dairy product consumption to the apparent inflammation in my joints causing me pain. I had been watching with interest the data being published on the potential hazards of giving children cow's milk very early in life with the development of autoimmune diseases, but I did not think about my own situation. If casein (milk protein) can potentially contribute to an immune response leading to diseases such as asthma and type 1 diabetes, couldn't it also be responsible for my joint pain? Apparently, it was; I have not had any more joint pain since I started the diet over three years ago!

I share my story with you to illustrate how even those in the field of nutrition, pharmaceuticals, and medicine can become so wrapped up in their own lives that they can lose touch with important new information and its correlation to their own health. To some extent, we are all asleep at the wheel regarding our health. It is time to wake up and face the fact that we will not have long, healthy lives nor will our children and grandchildren if we don't start paying at least as much attention to our nutrition and health as we do to gas prices!

Most importantly, I want to be clear that you do not have to be a dietitian in order to be successful. All you need to do is ignore all of the pop culture self-proclaimed nutrition experts who only serve to confuse you with their fads, and focus on incorporating what we know from valid science and well-conducted epidemiology studies into your daily nutrition habits. This book will help you do just that.

VEGANISM

· ·

What Is Veganism?

The vegan diet is simply one in which only plant-based foods are consumed. No animal products (meats) are eaten, including dairy and eggs. (The term is not synonymous with the word *vegetarian*, as vegetarians may eat dairy and eggs.) It is best to consume a wide variety of fruits, vegetables, grains, and legumes to help ensure you receive optimal nutrition. We will discuss this in more detail later. If you do add fat to your diet, it should be only in modest quantities of foods or oils containing relatively high omega-3 fatty acids, examples include canola and flaxseed oils.

Many books have been written on the subject of veganism. Compassionate people who feel that eating meat is wrong wrote most of these books. While I admire and applaud their convictions, that is not the intent of this book. Rather, this book is intended to help you live a more compassionate life for the best reason of all: your health!

Why Vegan?

Let me first be very clear: this book is not intended to exhaustively examine all of the research and science behind the advantages of the vegan diet. There are plenty of other books on the market that do a marvelous job of getting deeper into the science of plant-based nutrition. In fact, you have probably already bought into being plant-based for better health before you picked this book up. In this section, my aim is simply to enhance your commitment to follow a plant-based diet. What you will learn in this book is very much worth your time and effort. It will provide real-life how-tos, with the intention of leaving nothing to doubt. I will also give you some additional reasons to consider striving to move toward having a diet that is plant-based.

The other goal in this chapter is to show you why it makes no sense to buy into fads that focus on a single nutrient. They only create trouble. For example, a recent fad is to try to avoid carbohydrate since "carbs are bad." However, a plant-based diet is higher in carbohydrate, yet there are huge health advantages to it. Think about this: if the world's most renowned scientists have difficulty proving their nutritional theories because of the multiple factors that "dirty" their data, then why would we believe hucksters who have no data, manipulated data, or have made quantum leaps in logic based on limited data? This is exactly what happens when our society jumps on a fad, such as cutting out carbohydrate to extremes. In fact, it is quite difficult to study nutrition in human beings. Why? Because it is nearly impossible to isolate any one nutrient in our varied diet. That makes it nearly impossible to demonstrate cause and effect of any one nutrient as the reason for a change in health status. Let's consider an example. Recently, a friend told me that since he had switched to mostly whole grain pasta and bread products, his triglyceride level had come down quite a bit. He attributed the effect to the fact that he switched to whole grain products (the cause). I then asked him if he had become more conscious in general about his carbohydrate intake. "Oh yeah," he said. "My doctor told me I need to stay away from carbs."

"So your carb intake has gone down at the same time you switched to whole grain products?" I asked.

"Definitely," he said.

I went on to explain to him that excessive carbohydrate intake can cause triglycerides to become elevated because when the body has more carb than it needs for its current energy needs and glycogen storage, it converts what is left over to fat. Fat is stored in the body as triglyceride. The fact that he both reduced his intake of carbohydrate and switched over to whole grain at the same time makes it scientifically impossible to conclude that switching to whole grains alone caused his triglyceride level to decline. How can two changes at the same time be studied and an accurate conclusion be drawn? It can't usually be done with complete certainty. In fact, from a biochemical point of view, it is more likely that the reduction in triglycerides was due to the fact that he reduced his overall intake of carb and only partly due to the fact that he switched to whole grains.

Don't get me wrong; it is a very good thing for us all to move toward ditching the refined carbs for whole grain, but if the total amount of carbohydrate in the diet remains the same, it is unlikely to have an appreciable benefit in reducing triglycerides.

This example is just a simple illustration of how those without a solid science background can come to illogical conclusions about nutrition. This is a very intelligent man, but he is not a scientist.

There are hundreds of thousands of examples like this one out there. Just pick up any article or book on nutrition written by a layperson. The point is: we want you to start to think like a scientist so that you will not be fooled by the false prophets of nutritional claims.

Can you see why it is very difficult to study nutrition in human beings? There are just too many variables, including that person's genetic makeup, the environmental chemicals he or she is exposed to, the amount and type of stress in his or her life, the medicine he or she takes, and the hundreds of thousands of vitamins, minerals, phytochemicals, hormones, and pesticides in his or her food to come to a rational, scientific conclusion about any one nutrient in his or her diet.

In science, one example is called a case study, and it is not good science, just an anecdotal report. There are more rational approaches to better understand the role of nutrition in humans. For example, epidemiological studies in which thousands of people in a geographic location are studied and compared to people in a different geographical location allows for more appropriate cause and effect-like conclusions. Better yet, if other factors can be controlled for, such as genetics and environmental pollutants, it makes the conclusions even more reliable. For example, if the genetic makeup and environmental toxins of the people are very similar, then the differences observed from a nutritional variable are more likely to be real. This is why the results of *The China Study* were so valuable. The genetics and environmental toxins of the people studied were so similar that the differences between their results were most likely due to nutritional variables. Case studies are helpful in shedding light on subjects no one may be actively researching but should once there are enough case studies to signal a trend.

Laboratory studies conducted in proven animal models can also reliably predict effects on humans. The reason for this is that most factors that can influence the study results can usually be controlled: genetic makeup, environmental toxins, level of physical activity, and each and every nutrient the animal eats including the quantity of the nutrient being studied. For example, suppose I have one group of genetically similar rats whom I feed a diet which consists of 20 percent protein from casein (milk protein), then another group eating a diet containing 40 percent casein, and yet another containing 80 percent casein. The rest of the diets have exactly the same ingredients: rice and canola oil (albeit different percentages to make up the same amount of calories for each group of rats). The differences I observe in these rats would be most likely attributable to the levels of casein in the diet because to the best of my ability, I have controlled for all other factors. This is the good type of science that is very difficult to conduct in humans. This is why epidemiological studies in humans are so important. It studies large populations of people and identifies *tendencies* based on their lifestyle or exposure to other environmental entities.

Although some people snub animal studies, stating that whatever was studied has not been proven in humans, animal studies *are* very valuable, when the animal model itself has been proven to be a reliable model for whatever is being studied. Also, animals have a much shorter lifespan; thus, many generations can be studied in a relatively short period. Identifying potential carcinogens or other hazards in an animal model and then studying the effects in future generations can be predictive of the effects in humans; we just can't study it in humans within our own lifetime due to our lifespan. In addition, if a substance is suspected to be carcinogenic, it could not ethically be studied in a clinical trial in humans.

So what do we do when different studies produce different results? A rational approach is to weigh the evidence of the studies conducted, giving higher weight to those studies with higher scientific value (we will discuss this further in Part 5). Then connect the dots as logically as possible, and come to the most rational conclusion possible given the data studied. Fortunately, there have been so many well-conducted studies with consistent results when it comes to the benefit of the vegan diet with respect to our chronic diseases that we can safely conclude its many benefits.

The health benefits of vegan diets include lowering markers for cardiovascular disease and diabetes, improved bone health, and lowering the risk for many types of cancer.[1, 2, 3] In addition, a whole new science, called *nutrigenomics*, is arising. This science depicts how food and nutrition can turn on and off certain gene expression. For example, Japan has historically had very low rates of colorectal cancer in relation to the rates seen in the United States. While their diets do include some meat (mostly fish), they also contain significantly higher quantities of plant-based foods. However, when Japanese people migrate from Japan to the United States and begin consuming a more Western diet, their rate of colorectal cancer increases significantly.[4] In fact, the rate of colorectal cancer in Japan is now increasing with the increasing Westernization of the diet in Japan.[5] Similar observations have been made in populations of people with a traditionally low incidence of type 2 diabetes who consume a higher quantity of plant-based foods in their culture, then moving to a Westernized culture and subsequently developing diabetes.[6]

The genetic makeup for the tendency for developing cancer or diabetes did not change; what changed was the actual expression of these genes following chronic exposure to high fat, low fiber, and high animal protein of the Western diet. Think of the genes responsible for creating cancer as a light bulb in your house, and think of what you eat as a light switch. The light bulb is always there, but it only lights up when you flip the switch.

> Myth: Only things like radiation and nuclear waste affect our genes.

> Fact: Simple nutrition can affect whether certain genes "turn on."

The light goes off when you flip the switch in reverse. The same has shown to be true with hereditary diseases and nutrition. A person may have the gene(s) identified to lead to diseases like cancer, diabetes, and heart disease, but they have the ability to largely control whether those diseases switch on through what they eat. For example, Caitlin was diagnosed as insulin-resistant at age 13, but with an improved diet and exercise, her blood sugar levels and A1c are now within a normal range. Highly meat-based diets, which are subsequently high in saturated fat, highly processed foods, and low intake of fruits and vegetables, as well as generally higher in calories, can turn that switch on. The vegan diet can help turn the switch off.

In fact, it would take this entire book and many more volumes to share all of the scientific data that point in the direction of plant-based diets being the most nutrigenomically friendly. And while vegans may need to supplement some nutrients, such as vitamin B_{12}, iron, calcium, vitamin D, and perhaps omega-3 fatty acids, it is a small price to pay to prevent the horrors of cancer, diabetes, and cardiovascular disease! And in fact, as you will see in the supplementation chapter, even non-vegans in America are deficient in these nutrients. To date, the only treatment proven to reverse cardiac disease is a low fat vegan diet.[3] No drug has been proven to do exactly what the vegan diet has been shown to accomplish. And since cardiac disease is the #1 killer of the Western population, wouldn't it be silly not to investigate further the only treatment proven to reverse it while also preventing other chronic diseases?

For those of you who are concerned that a vegan diet would not have sufficient protein to meet your needs, there is good news. It is the position of the American Dietetic Association and Dietitians of Canada (now called the Academy of Nutrition and Dietetics) that a well-planned vegan diet is appropriate for all stages of life, including during pregnancy, lactation, infancy, childhood, and adolescence.[7] The association reviewed comparisons of the nutrient contents from the vegetarian, non-vegetarian (meat-eating), and vegan diets from many scientifically credible sources and came to its final position. Importantly, the association also concluded that isolated soy protein can meet our protein needs as effectively as animal protein, and is adequate to ensure we receive enough essential amino acids for growth and tissue repair. This should be great news for anyone concerned about getting adequate protein on a vegan diet!

There are other advantages to moving toward veganism besides the nutritional aspect. For one thing, if you have problems with constipation, know that your fiber intake is going to increase quite a bit, which should help alleviate quite a bit of this. You will also most likely find that you just feel better overall. You won't have that sluggishness you often get after a heavy meat meal. You will feel lighter. You may find those previous aches and pains are no longer there. Things on the inside are just functioning better.

Then there is the psychological benefit of knowing that what you are putting into your body is so much healthier than your previous diet. But let's also note here that not only should you move toward being vegan, but you should also strive to make your food choices whole foods. This means that to the best of your ability, you should stay away from refined foods.

> Myth: Any vegan diet is healthy.
>
> Fact: White bread and peanut butter alone are vegan, but eating just those would not be healthy. A variety of plants, grains, legumes/ seeds, and fruits are what makes for a healthy vegan diet.

An example of this is bread. You might determine that there are no animal products in a loaf of bread you pick up in the grocery store, but if it is white bread and not whole grain, you likely have not chosen the best product for your health. If you are not in the habit of choosing the more healthful products, fear not, for this will become second nature to you in a few months.

Another benefit is just how wonderful vegan meals can be. Many vegan recipes have incredibly creative uses of various herbs and spices, such that you may wonder where this food has been all your life. You won't miss the fat once you see how delicious meals can be without it. You will look forward to cooking, knowing that what you are making will be incredibly tasty as well as healthy.

This brings me to another point. Most of us have little time to cook healthful meals. That is just a fact. However, since you won't be cooking with meat, you will find that many of the dishes you make freeze really well. I usually take one day a month to make all of my seitan (vegan meats) and then store it in my freezer. That actually saves me time that I used to spend in the grocery store three or four times in a month to buy fresh meat. You can also make or buy whole grain breads and cook dried beans and store them in the freezer at the same time. You can buy frozen vegetables to complement the meals, and you should be set. Then you can complement what you have stored with fresh fruits, vegetables, and low fat desserts to feed your family. Are you beginning to see how there is no excuse to not try going vegan?

Another thing I found is that when your diet is almost completely plant-based, nothing has to go to waste. If you have the ability to have even a small composter, any scraps can be tossed in the composter for later use as fertilizer. I have been nothing short of amazed at the quality of the fertilizer we make at our house and how much money I have saved buying plant food!

By moving from a meat-based to a plant-based diet, you will reduce your eco-footprint on the environment. You will be going green. By reducing the amount of energy needed to raise animals for food, you will reduce the inevitable environmental pollutants generated both by the process of raising the animals, as well as reduce the quantities of pollutants released from these animals themselves.

Lastly, while you may not be thinking initially about being plant-based to avoid supporting animal cruelty, you may find, as I did, that it becomes a bigger part of your psyche than it was to start with. I can no longer pass by the meat section of a grocery store without thinking about what went in to providing that bloody piece of meat in the refrigerator. Animal cruelty was not the initial reason I went 95% vegan, but it is a motivator whenever I think back to the days of my eating meat. I just can't imagine putting any animal (other than fish, more on that later) in my mouth anymore.

> Myth: You will always crave your favorite meat or dairy product.
>
> Fact: Once you give the meat and dairy habit up for several months, they may not taste as good as they used to or as good as you remembered.

So by going to a plant-based diet, you will improve your health status, eat more delicious meals, potentially spend less time on grocery shopping and food preparation, make your own plant food, help save the planet, and avoid contributing to animal cruelty. Now can you think of any reason why you wouldn't want to strive to move in that direction?

You may be asking yourself how you can survive being vegan in a culture that still values meat as the primary basis for most meals. How will you handle dining out, going to other people's homes for dinner, finding a nutritious meal in a hurry if you are out and about? The answer is that when there is a will, there is a way. In addition, you can use non-vegan days as we will discuss on holidays and times when you absolutely have no choice but to eat animal-based products. While we will share many hints and tips, the truth is that most of the work figuring this part out will come from you. You will have to do some investigating in your own reality. We live in a major city where there is an abundance of options. You may live in a small town without all of the options accessible to us. We will teach you what you need to do, but we can't necessarily teach you exactly how to do it within your own reality. That will take some effort on your part, but we promise you that it can be done!

Why 95% Vegan?

Along the road of veganism, I realized that depending upon where I traveled, it was sometimes difficult to find pure vegan fare. It can be done, but only if the travel was either planned well in advance or if I had the time to access a local market that had an adequate selection for a vegan diet. Sometimes neither of the two was possible. Once I recognized this reality and lived with it as a busy road warrior, I came to the conclusion that rather than allow The Guilt Factor (TGF) to throw me off-track, I would figure out how to be 95% vegan. In science, a 5% difference is the usual wiggle room we give ourselves before we consider the variance to be significant, so why not apply this to my own reality? That is how the 95% vegan concept was born.

Before we go on with this discussion, let me reiterate that I am not suggesting that it wouldn't be wonderful if you could become 100% vegan, with no added fat. However, I also know based on my experience helping patients reduce their weight and otherwise improve their health status that demanding perfection can be cruel and dangerous. I remember with horror how I administered the old ADA diets to diabetic patients and told them that they could no longer have the foods that their entire lives revolved around. Imagine being a twenty-seven-year-old female patient raised in the South eating cheese grits every day for breakfast being told she didn't have enough fat exchanges in the day to be able to continue enjoying what she loved at least some of the time. It was cruel and certainly not something that patient could adhere to. Thus, it set the patient up for failure from the start, and I wasn't helping that patient be successful in managing her diabetes. To be clear, I didn't enjoy doing this to patients, but the ADA diet was the standard of care at the time. Thank goodness we have come a long way since then!

On the other hand, it would be irresponsible and ineffective for me not to provide you guidance with a goal in mind in order to improve your health status. You will not hear me say, "Everything in moderation." Nope, that isn't good enough. In the first place, what you consider to be moderation might be deadly. For example, you might believe that smoking ten cigarettes a day is moderate. However, over time, that smoking is putting you at a greater risk for developing COPD (Chronic Obstructive Pulmonary Disease, such as emphysema or chronic bronchitis), cardiovascular disease, and lung cancer. In this case, moderation can be deadly. Secondly, no one is ever successful without making a conscious effort and having a goal in mind.

Also to be clear, just as I pointed out in the introduction to the book that we don't know if the patients studied in *Preventing and Reversing Heart Disease*[1] could have been just as successful being less vegan with some added fat, I have not conducted any formal scientific studies on the 95% Vegan plan. However, I do know how people are not successful in general, and that is when they try to implement extreme changes they cannot adhere to long-term. I will help you and your family to be very successful in attaining a healthy weight and prevent heart disease, cancer, and diabetes. The way to do that is to provide you a plan that is more realistic so you can stick to it for the long haul.

The other reality to keep in mind is how much more successful you will be by the numbers if you are consistently striving toward a 95% goal versus trying and failing a number of times by trying to adhere to a diet that is not as user friendly for more than a couple of weeks. I will warn you that we are about to get into some math right now. Please do not be concerned that you will have to do complicated math in order to be successful. You will not. Remember, the premise of this concept is that you do not have to be perfect. I am simply going through an example in fine detail to illustrate my point while also helping you cut through the bull, as it were. Let's take a look at a forty-year-old man, 5'11", and weighing two hundred pounds. His body mass index (BMI) is 27.9, which is considered overweight. Not obese, mind you, just overweight (a BMI of 30 or greater is considered obese, more to come on this later). In order to maintain his weight at two hundred pounds, this man of light activity must consume, on average, around 2,700 calories daily.[2] Let's take a look at this man's typical daily eating pattern to see how he achieves maintaining a weight of 200 lb[3]:

	Portion Size	Calories	Grams of Fat	Grams of Total Carbohydrate	Grams of Protein
Breakfast					
Raisin bran	1 cup	195	2	47	5
Skim milk	1 cup	83	0	12	8
Orange juice	1/2 cup	56	0	13	1
Half-and-half for coffee	1/4 cup	79	7	3	2
Lunch					
Roast Beef	3 oz	121	2	0	23
American cheese	2 oz	179	12	6	9
Sub roll	1 small	250	1	52	9
Mayonnaise	1 oz	196	22	0	0
Potato chips	1 small bag	152	10	15	2
Brownie	2 oz	237	13	30	3
Snack					
Crackers from vending machine	1 pack	180	9	16	6
Half-and-half for afternoon coffee	1/4 cup	79	7	3	2

	Portion Size	Calories	Grams of Fat	Grams of Total Carbohydrate	Grams of Protein
Dinner					
Grilled chicken	6 oz	180	3	0	36
Mashed potatoes	4 oz	128	5	19	2
Green peas	1 cup	134	0	25	9
Dinner roll	1 oz	76	2	13	2
Butter for roll and vegetables	1 Tbsp	102	12	0	0
Snack					
Vanilla ice cream	1 cup	289	16	34	5
Totals		2716	123	288	124
Calories ratio			41%	42%	18%

It is no surprise that the example looks like the typical American diet. While it doesn't appear to be extreme, this diet is causing this man to be about twenty-five pounds overweight. Also notice that the percentage of calories from fat in his current diet is around 41. This is also typical of the Westernized diet that is killing us.

Now, let's say this man decides he wants to lose this weight very quickly. He decides he is going to go on a low carbohydrate diet. After all, he can eat all of the bacon and other meat he wants since it has no carbs. All he has to do is keep his carbs down to thirty grams per day. Here is an example of a typical day while he is following this diet:

	Portion Size	Calories	Grams of Fat	Grams of Total Carbohydrate	Grams of Protein
Breakfast					
Bacon	4 slices	168	13	0	12
Eggs, fried	2 eggs	199	15	2	13
American cheese	2 oz	179	12	6	9
Half-and-half for coffee	1/4 cup	79	7	3	2
Lunch					
Roast Beef	6 oz	242	4	0	46
American cheese	2 oz	179	12	6	9
Iceberg lettuce	2 oz	8	0	2	1
Snack					
Turkey	3 oz	115	1	0	26
Half-and-half for coffee	1/4 cup	79	7	3	2
Dinner					
Ribeye Steak	8 oz	578	45	0	43
Iceberg lettuce	2 oz	8	0	2	1
Tomato	2 oz	27	0	4	2

	Portion Size	Calories	Grams of Fat	Grams of Total Carbohydrate	Grams of Protein
Snack					
Eggs, fried	2 eggs	199	15	2	13
Totals		2060	131	30	179
Calories ratio			57%	6%	35%

Although he is eating what seems like a feast every day, he has actually cut his daily food intake by 656 calories. But look at the fact that his total intake is almost 57 percent from fat! Does this seem healthy? And since there are approximately 3,500 calories per pound of body weight, this man would lose over a pound per week, over the long haul, whether or not he restricted his carb intake. However, when we severely restrict carbohydrate, our bodies lose water at a fast rate, so the initial rate of weight loss is even greater[4], leading us to believe it is a miracle diet. It isn't. It has you peeing your brains out as you starve your body from carb, and it is rapidly breaking down glycogen, fat, and even muscle tissue to feed itself. It is producing acidic ketones that can be toxic to body organs. Also, your brain must have carbohydrate as an energy source. The breakdown of fat is not giving the brain what it needs for a ready energy source.

The reality of any diet that enables weight loss is that it is providing fewer calories than one needs to maintain their current weight. Whatever the scheme, the reality is that the diet has you eating fewer calories than you need to maintain your current weight. The number of calories you need to maintain your current weight depends on how much you currently weigh, your age, your gender, your height, the amount of stress and physical activity you have. Anything less than that will create a negative calorie balance, resulting in weight loss. Since one pound of fat is equivalent to 3,500 calories, if you cut back by 500 calories per day, you will lose one pound per week. Cutting out 1,000 calories per day will cause you to lose two pounds per week and so on.

Calories are only derived from protein, carbohydrate, and fat. Salt does not provide calories. If your kidneys don't clear the salt (sodium) well from the blood, it will cause you to retain water. This has led many people to believe that salt can cause weight gain. It only does this by causing you to retain water, not by creating more fat in your body. However, it is still a good idea to limit your salt intake as it can raise your blood pressure if you are not clearing the sodium well.

So this gentleman thinks he is doing great, for about three weeks. He has lost fifteen pounds, and his clothes are fitting much better. Everyone around him comments about how great he looks, and he tells them it's all because of this low carb diet he has been on.

The problem is, he has these carb cravings that are driving him crazy. He hasn't eaten any pasta, bread, or starchy vegetables. No milk or cereal either. He walks past an Italian restaurant, and the aroma makes his mouth water. He thinks, "Just a little pasta won't set me back too much." So he eats a plate of spaghetti for dinner that night. He feels so good, and the spaghetti was so delicious.

Then, usually one of two things happens—either he feels guilty for going off his diet or he realizes just how deprived he has been. In either case, he eventually winds up as heavy as he was before or perhaps worse. He binges on carbs for a week, does well for a couple of days, but decides he just can't stick to the low carb diet anymore. This is a typical example for why people say, "I was on the (fill-in-the-blank) diet for a while," the key word being *was*. In short, he gives up on himself for a while. He teeters between his usual diet and attempts to stick to the low carb diet for another year, then another. It should be very obvious to you that this is not a healthy way to live, especially considering his overall fat intake both before and during the low carb diet.

The success rate for obese people losing 10 percent of their body weight and not regaining it for over five years is around 20 percent.[5] That is the best-case scenario. More commonly, people follow a pattern similar to the gentleman described above and stay overweight or climb into the obesity statistic. We want to increase that success rate through a healthy approach that is doable for the long haul.

Let's also realize that in the example above, the man's fat intake, mostly saturated fat, was anywhere from 41 percent to 57 percent. Is it any wonder that he was headed for trouble from a health perspective? It's anyone's guess as to how soon that first heart attack will occur.

Now let's take a look at the same scenario, but instead of the man trying a low carb diet to lose weight in order to look good, he strives to be 95% vegan. When I say 95% vegan, I mean that 95 percent of the overall diet's calories come from plant sources. The other 5 percent of calories can come from animal sources: meat and dairy. As for me, I never eat anything with a foot (including hooves and claws). I stick with fins (fish) when there aren't enough vegan options because there exists enough reliable data around the value of fish in the diet for me to worry about adding it to my diet every now and then. Also, the amount of fish I could possibly consume at 5 percent of my total calories does not have me concerned about mercury poisoning either. I may have dairy and eggs *very* occasionally when I travel, if there is not an adequate supply of vegan options. I successfully maintain a 95% vegan status overall. You can too, easily.

Let's get back to our gentleman. Let's look at three different days of possible dietary intake, two that are 100% vegan and the other where he incorporates animal products. This will help you see how you can easily achieve 95% vegan without having to work any calculations for yourself. Note that the gentleman read all of the food labels to determine that each product is 100% plant-based (we will discuss how to do this in Part 3).

100% vegan day 1 (cited recipes are reprinted with permission in Appendix 2):

	Portion Size	Calories	Grams of Fat	Grams of Total Carbohydrate	Grams of Protein
Breakfast					
Raisin bran	1 cup	195	2	47	5
Light vanilla soy milk	1 cup	69	1	7	6
Orange juice	1/2 cup	56	0	13	1
Soy Creamer for Coffee	1/4 cup	60	4	4	0
Snack					
Organic apple	1 large	110	0	29	1
Lunch					
Hummus- store bought individual container	1 container	150	13	7	3
Whole grain crackers	6 crackers	103	3	19	3
Assorted steamed vegetables (all non-starchy)	2 cups	88	1	16	10
Snack					
Dried cherries	1-1/2 oz	138	0	35	0
Soy Creamer for Coffee	1/4 cup	60	4	4	0
Dinner					
Seitan cutlets (vegan meat)*	2 servings	233	5	10	38
Green peas	1 cup	134	0	25	9

	Portion Size	Calories	Grams of Fat	Grams of Total Carbohydrate	Grams of Protein
Baked potato	1 medium	168	0	37	5
Steamed yellow squash	1 cup	18	0	3	2
Fresh peach	1 medium	38	0	9	1
Snack					
Rice Dream® frozen dessert	1 serving	140	6	22	0
Totals		1760	39	287	84
Calories ratio			20%	65%	19%

* Seitan cutlet recipe is from *Veganomicon*, by Isa Chandra Moskowitz and Terry Hope Romero (2007), pg 132. ISBN-13: 978-1-56924-264-3

Let's analyze the facts from 100% vegan day 1. Our gentleman's caloric intake is now around 1,760, cutting approximately 1,000 calories from the amount of calories it takes to maintain his unhealthy weight. Cutting 1,000 calories per day will allow him to lose two pounds per week, whether or not he is exercising. He could lose that extra twenty-five pounds within thirteen weeks. But just look at the food content for the day. It allows for his previous indulgences, in that he is still allowing for coffee creamer (just not cow's milk-based) a large quantity of food at dinner and a sweet treat before bedtime. However, the new improved diet has him consuming more than ten servings of fruits and vegetables on this day and has also cut this man's fat intake to 20 percent down from 41 to 57 percent! Best of all, he has had no intake of saturated fat or meat protein at all yet plenty of protein. Who could argue that this is not a superior approach to what he previously tried in order to lose weight?

Let's look at what day 2 of 100% vegan might look like. For this example day, let's pretend that our gentleman does this for one day over his weekend.

	Portion Size	Calories	Grams of Fat	Grams of Total Carbohydrate	Grams of Protein
Breakfast					
Southwest tofu scramble*	1 serving	118	5	7	12
Tempeh bacon**	1 serving	124	6	5	10
Orange juice	1/2 cup	56	0	13	1
Soy Creamer for Coffee	1/4 cup	60	4	4	0
Whole wheat toast	2 slices	138	2	26	5
Strawberry preserves	1 oz	71	0	18	0
Snack					
Dried apricots	1-1/2 oz.	120	0	29	1
Lunch					
Hummus, commercially prepared	2 oz	162	12	6	2
Whole grain crackers	6 crackers	103	3	19	3
Assorted steamed vegetables (all non-starchy)	2 cups	88	1	16	10
Snack					
Vegan oatmeal raisin cookies***	2 cookies	242	8	40	4
Soy Creamer for Coffee	1/4 cup	60	4	4	0
Dinner					
Pasta, cooked	10 oz	352	3	71	12
Spinach, cooked	1 cup	41	0	7	5
Tomato sauce	1 cup	220	12	22	4
TVP meatballs****	4 balls	190	6	19	29

	Portion Size	Calories	Grams of Fat	Grams of Total Carbohydrate	Grams of Protein
Snack					
Vegan Rice Pudding	1 serving with raisins	346	1	50	7
Totals		2491	67	356	105
Calories ratio			24%	57%	17%

* Southwest Tofu Scramble recipe is from *The 30 Minute Vegan*, by Mark Reinfeld and Jennifer Murray (2009), pp 62-63, published by Da Capo Press, a member of the Perseus Books Group. ISBN-13: 978-0-7832-1327-9

** Tempeh Bacon recipe is from *Vegan Brunch*, by Isa Chandra Moskowitz (2009), pg 141,Published by Da Capo Press, a member of the Perseus Books Group. ISBN: 978-0-7382-1272-2.

*** Oatmeal Raisin Cookie recipe is from *Vegan Cookies Invade Your Cookie Jar*, by Isa Chandra Moskowitz and Terry Hope Romero (2009), pg 75, published by Da Capo Press, a member of the Perseus Books Group. ISBN:978-1-60094-048-4

**** TVP is Texturized Vegetable Protein, available at many grocery stores. Pour 1 cup boiling water over 1 cup granules and let stand. Mix in any seasonings you want and use as ground beef. This example assumes the meatballs were made with 2 cups TVP, 2 cups boiling water, and 1 Tbsp oil. Recipe made 12 meatballs.

***** Vegan Rice Pudding recipe is Reprinted from *The Vegan Diner*, by Jule Hasson. Available from Running Press, an imprint of The Perseus Books Group. Copyright © 2011.

So this day isn't quite as stellar as his typical working day, but like all of us, he isn't perfect. He is trying though, and he is still only getting 24 percent of his calories from fat, no animal products, and is still consuming fewer calories than previously. This day was full of nutrients, including fiber.

Now, let's take a look at what his day might look like when he is permitting himself to have meat (day 3). Since he no longer has cow's milk in the refrigerator and has adapted the rest of his pantry to represent that of a vegan, he continues to use non-animal-based products (e.g. soy milk). This third day example is something he allows himself sporadically throughout the year.

	Portion Size	Calories	Grams of Fat	Grams of Total Carbohydrate	Grams of Protein
Breakfast					
Raisin bran	1 cup	195	2	47	5
Light vanilla soy milk	1 cup	69	1	7	6
Soy Creamer for Coffee	1/4 cup	60	4	4	0
Orange juice	1/2 cup	56	0	13	1
Lunch					
Fresh ground honey peanut butter	3 Tbsp	269	19	12	10
Whole wheat bread	2 slices	138	2	26	5
Fresh Strawberries	1 cup	46	0	11	1
Dinner					
Ribeye Steak	8 oz	578	45	0	43
Baked potato	1 medium	168	0	37	5
Green salad	2 cups	0	0	0	0
Dinner roll	1 oz	76	2	13	2
Butter for roll and baked potato	1 Tbsp	102	12	0	0
Sour cream for baked potato	2 oz	77	6	4	2
Red wine	2 - 4oz glasses	198	0	6	0
Raspberry sorbet	3.4 cup	150	0	38	0

	Portion Size	Calories	Grams of Fat	Grams of Total Carbohydrate	Grams of Protein
Totals		2182	93	218	80
Calories ratio			38%	40%	15%
Percent of calories from animal-based food = 578 + 102+ 77/2182 = 35%					

So this day wasn't perfect either. Our gentleman enjoyed a night out to dinner with a steak and some wine. Still, his total calories were about five hundred less than what it took to maintain his previously unhealthy weight. The percent of calories from animal-based food for the day was 35 percent, and his percent of calories from fat approached his previous unhealthy diet.

Now, let's put this all into perspective mathematically, using these three days' values for demonstration purposes. I will go through the math with you, but please don't glaze over. I just want to illustrate how this works.

Let's assume this man's day 1 example became his typical day, for most days of the month, say twenty-five out of thirty. Day 2 became his typical day for one day of the week, for four days out of thirty. His day 3 (animal-based food) came sporadically but enough so that he never felt deprived. Let's say he decided he needed one day per month as day 3 in order to feel satiated and so that he can continue to socialize at meat-eating events without having to go to extraordinary means to stay healthy.

Day	Days per month	Calories per day	Calories per month	% Animal-Based Calories	Total Animal-Based Calories per month
1	25	1750	43750	0	0
2	4	2491	9964	0	0
3	1	2182	2182	35	764
Totals			55896		764

So if one day per month looked like day 3, his percent of animal-based calories would be

$$764/55{,}896 \times 100 = 1.4\%$$

He would be 98.6% vegan, even better than what he is striving for, in spite of eating meat one meal per month! This gives him some wiggle room in case he adds a few more meat-eating days during the year.

In addition, his total of 55,896 calories per month reduces his previous unhealthy calorie consumption by 25,584 (81,480 minus 55,896), which equates to seven pounds per month. Our gentleman will lose seven pounds per month, losing his twenty-five pounds in less than four months! This calculation does not take into account any exercise he might decide to start, which would permit him to lose the weight more quickly (and increase his muscle mass, which would boost his metabolism to burn even more calories per day).

The following table illustrates all of the days we discussed so that you can compare and contrast.

	Calories	Grams of Fat	Grams of Carb	Grams of Protein
The Old Diet	2716	123	288	124
The Low Carb Diet	2060	131	30	179
100% Vegan Day 1	1760	39	287	84
100% Vegan Day 2	2491	67	356	105
Meat Day for 95% Vegan	2182	93	218	80
95% Vegan - Monthly Weighted Averages*	1860	45	294	87
95% Vegan PERCENTAGES		22%	63%	15%
* These figures take into account the man is having 25 per month day 1, 4 days per months of Day 2, and 1 day per month from the meat-eating day				

Now for the really good news: our gentleman could actually have four animal-based meals per month, given the same proportions as in our example to be 95% vegan, roughly one meal per week! Now that sounds doable, doesn't it?

Here is the math, in case you are interested. If not, feel free to skip ahead to the next paragraph.

Assume there are 30 days in each month

If 4 days have one animal based meal, per the example of our gentleman, there are 26 days left in the month
To keep the same ratio of Day 1 and Day 2 for the total of 26 days:
25 days of Day 1
4 Days of Day 2
Equals 29 days total;
Therefore, for 26 days total, we would have 22 days of Day 1, and 4 days of Day 2

	Calories per Day	Total Days	Total Calories per 30 Days	Total Animal Based Calories	Total Animal Based Calories per 30 Days
Day 1	1760	22	38720	0	0
Day 2	2491	4	9964	0	0
Day 3	2182	4	8728	764	3056
Total per 30 Days			57412		3056
3056/57412 X 100 = 5.3% Rounded to 5%					

In this scenario, our gentleman would be losing close to the same amount of weight per month, so being 95% vegan versus 98.6 percent doesn't change his success in losing weight. Being 95% vegan has only upside potential from his previous lifestyle. It improves his risks to help avoid heart attack, stroke, diabetes, and certain types of cancer. It has him getting to his goal weight in less than six months. He is going green, living a more compassionate lifestyle. Yet he is not swearing off all animal products thereby setting him up for failure from the start.

This, ladies and gentlemen, is how it works. Your nutrition is a big picture over many months and years, not limited to how you feel about it in a moment, a day, or a week. So rather than sporadically taking up some fad diet to lose weight quickly in an unhealthy manner, doesn't it make sense to stop and think about your overall health? Doesn't it make sense to think more long-term and realize you don't have to be perfect to lose weight and improve your health status? I think so.

Our example gentleman is not a fluke. The math didn't work out by accident. We could look at any other person under the same scenario and come to the same conclusion. Their total number of calories needed may differ, but the overall proportion will remain the same. If only one meal per week consumed contains animal-based food, the calculations will still come very close to this one. If our example were a female, she would have correspondingly lower total calories, yet the percentage of contributing nutrients to her overall intake would be very similar to our gentleman. The bottom-line is that if your diet is plant-based for your entire food intake except one meal per week, you will be 95% vegan. We do not need to concern ourselves with protein or carbohydrate because adequate amounts of both will be consumed by eating a wide variety of foods. In fact, if you aren't adding fat to your diet and you are limiting your intake of nuts, olives, avocado, and other naturally occurring fat from plant sources, you really needn't concern yourself with your overall fat intake either. We will discuss these nutrients in more detail later.

If you are a person who likes to have a handle on exactly what you eat, the calories, grams of fat, etc. you can certainly do this. There are plenty of reference books out there with the nutritional content of many foods, often including restaurant food estimates.

One of my favorites is *Calorie King*[6]. It is quite inexpensive yet pretty much everything you need is there.

If you wish to calculate your fat intake by hand, including total percent of calories from fat, please see Appendix 3 to learn how to do this.

I promised earlier that you would not have to do math to get to 95% vegan, and you don't. You do not have to calculate calories or grams of fat. Your goals are very simple. You will strive to do the following:

1. Eat one meal per week (or less) containing animal based items.

2. You will rarely add fat, including having fried foods, and will limit your consumption of high fat-containing raw foods, such as nuts, olives, or avocados.

3. Eat as much whole food (versus processed) as possible.

4. Not allow TGF to throw you off from your progress

All that math brings us to one simple rule—to become 95% Vegan with three additional guidelines to ensure the highest quality, lowest guilt factor diet. As you move forward, remember you are striving to reach these goals. It will take some time to figure out how to cut out the fat and processed foods, so it is very important that you always remember guideline number 4. Make improvements every day, and don't give in to guilt if you aren't perfect.

Now, let's get to work!

THE IMPORTANCE OF LEARNING HOW TO FISH

· ·

Chinese Proverb:

If you give a man a fish you feed him for a day. If you teach a man to fish you feed him for a lifetime.

—Lao Tzu, 4th Century BC

The pregnant woman sitting before me had gestational diabetes. In most cases, gestational diabetes resolves after the baby is born, so our goal for that session was to teach her how to make it through the pregnancy full-term and have a healthy baby.

She was an intelligent woman, ready to learn, motivated by the precious baby growing inside her. So off I went, teaching her about how to manage her carb intake since it was extremely important that she tightly manage her postprandial (one and two hours after she ate a meal or snack) blood sugar. I used many examples from the foods she told me were important to her in order to provide what she needed, but in a controlled, mathematical way. After about forty-five minutes into my teaching, she just groaned, "Please, just tell me what to eat. I can do anything for the next five months!" I felt her pain. I switched over to just providing a strict diet for her to follow every day, and she was very happy.

Two weeks later, the same woman showed up in my office. "I can't stand eating the same things every day," she said. "Can we do something different?"

It was at that moment that I realized my approach with her initially was too much like a classroom lecture. Had I gotten her more involved, such as having her write out her own meal plan, based on the principles I taught her, she might not have gotten so frustrated. I could have broken the teaching into smaller pieces, ensuring she grasped each section by putting it into a plan that would fit her life. By making her more involved in the process, she might not have glazed over and begged me to just tell her what to eat.

In fact, actively engaging the student in the learning process provides a much greater retention rate.[1] You will likely not retain the teachings in this book without somehow being actively involved in your learning. Moreover, I would not be doing you any service by just telling you what to do. Rather, I will actively involve you in your own learning by providing suggested assignments, with all of the how-tos you will need. The great thing is that you can learn at your own pace; no one is watching you! Think of the homework exercises as a treasure hunt for your health. You owe it to yourself and your family to find the buried treasure that can help you lead a longer and much healthier life. You will recognize a suggested assignment by the heading Homework.

I urge you to keep notes about these homework assignments or make entries from the homework assignments into your copy of *The 95% Vegan Diet Workbook*. It may seem silly at first, but the information will prove useful to you in the future. In a year from now, you can review everything you did to take full control of your diet and your health and give yourself a good pat on the back.

Tell me and I will forget. Show me and I may remember. Involve me and I will understand.

—Chinese Proverb

CREATING A RIPPLE EFFECT, GENERATION-TO-GENERATION

· ·

Our Western diet is killing us, plain and simple. It has increased our weight dramatically over the last fifty years. In fact, from 1960–62 to 2005–06, the prevalence of obesity increased from 13.4 to 35.1 percent in US adults aged twenty to seventy-four.[1,2] That means that the prevalence of obesity in the United States has increased by more than 250 percent since 1960! Individuals who are obese have a significantly increased risk of early death from all causes, compared with healthy weight individuals (BMI 18.5 to 24.9). Most of the increased risk of death is due to cardiovascular disease (heart attack and stroke). There are over 112,000 excess deaths due to cardiovascular disease, over 15,000 excess deaths due to cancer, and over 35,000 excess deaths due to non-cancer, non-cardiovascular disease causes per year in the obese US population.[3]

At the same time our weight has increased, our meat consumption rose by about 200 percent[4], yet less than one in ten Americans achieves their recommended intake of fruit and vegetables.[5]

How in the world did this happen to us?

For those of you too young to know this, there was once a time when our parents put a scoop of each vegetable and a small portion of meat on our plates, and that was it. There were no second helpings. We didn't eat more than one dinner roll or biscuit for dinner. Our desserts were often just fruit. Ice cream was an every now-and-then treat. Our parents would tell us "no more" if they felt we had had enough of a particular food on the table. We did not starve. We were a healthy skinny. We were too busy playing outside to think much about food.

You can draw your own conclusions about why we have become such an overindulgent nation. Suffice it to say that we have clearly lost a healthy dose of self-control. But think about this: it has taken two generations for the statistics above to play out. While I do believe it will take time to reverse the horrible trends, if we start right now, we will likely come a long way in our own lifetime. So let's begin by setting some clear boundaries in which we can create a healthy ripple effect for the generations ahead. I have started a list of simple guidelines for parents and grandparents to help you. As you think about your own reality, you will likely create some guidelines and boundaries of your own. Mine are just the first ten:

The First Ten Guidelines to Create a Ripple Effect, Generation-to-Generation

1. Make the nutrition of your family a priority. Keep your vision for creating a nutritionally healthy environment top of mind for your kids. This will teach them that their health is something to be respected and cherished.

2. Make the physical activity of your family a priority. You don't have to have a gym membership to ensure your family is getting enough exercise. Play outside with your kids, jump rope, play tag, or whatever your child's preference. Take a stroll around the block with your kids when you all get home for the day. If you can't get outside where you live to exercise, explore what may be available in your community for you and your kids to do. This will allow

your kids to tell you about their day at the same time you are all getting some exercise in.

3. Teach your kids how to fish. Create a poster board for a daily nutrition roundup that actively engages them. However, you choose to do it; help them understand the importance of keeping their fat and animal protein intake low.

4. Take your kids to the supermarket or farmer's market and involve them in the selection of fresh fruits, vegetables, and whole grains. Encourage them to choose all of the different food colors so that they have a varied diet. If the fresh whole food is too expensive, take them over to the freezer section and select some less pricey options. Help them understand why choices are good or not. For example, is it too high in fat and too low in fiber? Does the product contain animal products?

5. Do not reward your kids with food. I cringe when I hear parents promising some fattening treat (such as a candy bar or ice cream) as a reward. Your kids will value even more highly rewards that involve spending time together doing something they will enjoy. For example, when your child brings home that A+ test, why not celebrate with a trip to the nearest playground? This will also give them and you some much-needed exercise.

6. Remember, you are in charge of your own wallet. If your kids beg you for an unhealthy fast-food meal, you do have a choice. Perhaps you can get them to think about how that money could be better spent, while reminding them the reasons why they are not going to eat that unhealthy meal. You might even start saving the money you would have spent in a jar at home and ultimately spend it on something much more enjoyable for the whole family. It is

always good to give your kids a visual when trying to teach them a principle.

7. Do not offer second helpings. We already eat far too much. Help your kids understand what a healthy portion size looks like, and tell them when they have had enough. This is just a boundary that children need to learn so that they will carry it through to adulthood.

8. Teach your children that it is okay to be hungry. For some reason, we have gotten to the point in our society where we think any pangs of hunger are unacceptable when in fact, they are normal. Think about how often you eat when you are not even hungry. Yes, there is a psychological component to feeling hungry, such as smelling food or seeing a commercial that makes your kids want to run out and grab that huge steak burger. This is another boundary that is healthy for children to learn: to have the self-discipline out of respect for their health to not succumb to the temptation to gorge themselves every time their tummies grumble a little bit.

9. Minimize trips to the local fast-food restaurants. Although some of them are trying to convince you they have healthier options, oftentimes they are adding items that may be a bit lower in fat (still too high, in some cases) but have large quantities of simple sugars—in short, not healthy options.

10. Address it quickly if your kids start to head down the wrong nutritional path. If they are being influenced by other kids to make unhealthy food or dietary habit choices, remind them of what they learned when they were out grocery shopping with you, as well as all of the other lessons you have weaved into their minds.

Above all this, *you* must become a role model for your children; *you* must also follow these guidelines. And as you incorporate these ten guidelines into your family's reality, you will come across so many best practices. Be sure to share them with others in your community and also learn from them. This is how we will find our way out of this unhealthy mess we have allowed to take over, by creating a ripple effect throughout our communities as well as from generation-to-generation!

PART 2:
First Things First

The timeless words of Thomas Edison were, "There is no substitute for hard work." If you are like most Americans, you have bought into any number of schemes to become healthier and lose weight. You bought products that promised to burn fat without you having to make an effort. You ate foods that people touted are fat-burning. You bought magazines and books that promised a miracle, whether it was weight loss, stamina, or the fountain of youth. You are certainly not alone. There are millions of other people who have done the same and who have been disappointed, over and over again, just like you.

We will address the fads and disappointing products in Part 5, as we learn to become our own scientists. For now, suffice it to say that there is no miracle product or food that will do any of the above-mentioned promises. In order to be successful, you are going to have to put in some needed work. But think about this: Wouldn't you rather put in some active work in one solid effort and be successful rather than put in minor, passive efforts over and over again that leave you disappointed and no healthier (but less wealthy) than before? Isn't it time to really think about what we have been doing and put a stop to it? If you agree, then read on. You are going to gain the knowledge you need to put in this one effort for the last time. Once you have read this book and completed the suggested assignments, you will be equipped with what you truly need to know to reverse the trend you have been on, likely for many years.

ASSESSING YOUR NUTRITIONAL HEALTH STATUS

· ·

Your overall health, including nutritional status, is based on a number of different parameters. You can assess some of these parameters yourself at home, while others are measured through blood samples. Whenever you begin any new diet or health program, it is a good idea to schedule a visit with your doctor so that he or she can draw these blood samples to determine your health status. These initial blood tests also provide you a baseline so that you can see during subsequent office visits how your diet is affecting your health.

Think of all of the fad diets that promise one thing or another, yet there were no recommendations of actual clinical measurements to point to in order to determine how it was truly impacting your internal health. How can anyone emphatically state that a diet, supplement, herbal remedy, or drug works without having valid measurements with which you would know the statement was true? The answer is, they can't. But now you are going to learn about the basic measurements you can follow to truly monitor your 95% vegan diet's effect on your health. You are going to take full control.

Before we get started, let me first state that the most important thing you can do for your health is to not smoke. All of the nutrition in the world cannot undo the damage from smoking. So step number 1 is to quit smoking, if you do smoke.

Likewise, if you have high blood pressure, you need to do whatever it takes to get it under control. Weight loss, exercise, and decreased salt intake can all help, but many people will still need medicine, sometimes two, three, or more different types of medications to achieve the recommended target. As you lose weight, the dosages of your medications will likely decline, and you may even be able to stop taking some of them. However, I cannot stress strongly enough that there is no shame in taking medication to control your blood pressure. Not taking medication when you know better and then suffering a heart attack or stroke is cause for shame. Most importantly, know what your targets are for your blood pressure. If you don't have targets that are based in evidence-based medicine, how will you know you are at an optimal state? For most people, the target will be less than 130/85, but some people need an even lower target. Again, please partner with your physician to make the right decisions for you.

Appendix 4 provides a means for you to record and track the elements of your health status. Note that your physician will not likely check all of the blood levels listed at each office visit. This is okay, but do be sure to ask for a test if you feel you need to have it done.

HOME BASED ASSESSMENTS FOR NUTRITIONAL HEALTH STATUS

Did you know that obesity is actually considered a form of malnutrition? We usually think of malnutrition in terms of wasting away from starvation. However, malnutrition simply means "bad nutrition," and obesity is certainly an example!

There are a few different ways of assessing if we suffer from the malnutrition of being overweight or obese.

First, we consider a person's body mass index (BMI). It is a means to look at your weight, relative to your height, to determine if you are carrying any excess pounds. In most cases, excess pounds come in the form of fat. However, in some cases, such as in athletes, excess pounds can be in the form of muscle. Also, if a person has a large frame, meaning heavy bones, some excess weight can be in the bone structure. In these cases, BMI may not be an indicator of being overweight. You know your own body, so try to objectively assess if BMI would be an accurate assessment of your weight status. For example, if you know you have "love handles," a "spare tire," or a big behind, then BMI is likely going to be a useful tool for you.

BMI, combined with your waist measurement, almost always provides a clear picture of your overweight status. To calculate your BMI, you can use an online calculator, such as is availa-

ble on the CDC website: http://www.cdc.gov/healthyweight/
assessing/bmi

You can also calculate your BMI using this equation:

[Weight in pounds ÷ (height in inches × height in inches)]
× 703

or if you prefer to calculate in metric:

Weight in kilograms ÷ (height in meters × height in
meters)

For example, if a person weighs 200 pounds (90.9 kg) and is 5
feet, 6 inches (1.68 meters) tall, the calculation would be:

Using pounds and inches:

200 ÷ (66 × 66) × 703 = 32.3

Using metric measurements:

90.9 ÷ (1.68 × 1.68) = 32.5

Normal BMI ranges from 18.5 to 24.9, overweight BMI
ranges from 25.0 to 29.9, class I obesity ranges from 30.0 to 34.9,
class II obesity ranges from 35.0 to 39.9, and extreme obesity is
a BMI of 40 or above. In the case above, with a BMI of 32.3, the
person would be considered obese class I.

If there is a question of whether BMI is an accurate assessment of weight status, you can measure your waist circumference.
To do this, place a tape measure around your abdomen above the
hip bones (iliac crests) and over the umbilicus (belly button), as
illustrated in figure 1 below. Do not make the tape measure so
tight that it indents your skin. Visually check to make sure the
tape is at an even height all the way around. For women, if the
measurement is 31-½ inches or greater, that would signal that
the BMI measurement is likely an accurate depiction of weight
status. For men, the waist measurement of 37 or above would
be a signal that the BMI measurement is an accurate depiction

of weight status. I can't tell you how many patients and people I have spoken to who are critical of BMI and don't think it is appropriate for them. However, the fact is that BMI is appropriate for the majority of people; most simply do not want to face it. You would have to be *extremely* muscular or have an obviously large frame for it not to work for you.

Figure 1

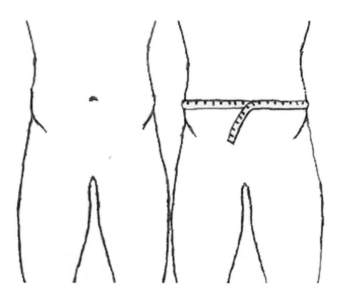

BMI status and waist circumference used together almost always provide an accurate picture for a person's risk for hypertension, type 2 diabetes, some cancers[1], and blood lipid (fat) abnormalities[2]—all consequences of being overweight. And although the literature cites varying measurements that signal certain increases in risk status for cardiovascular disease, diabetes, colon, and breast cancer, it is safe to say in general that the greater the waist measurement, the greater the risk.

Body fat measurement is also indicative of overweight/obesity status. However, it is more difficult to ascertain this number, and there are no solid guidelines for what your percentage of body fat should be.[3] Healthy percentages appear to vary and are dependent on other variables, such as sex and ethnicity. There are several ways in which your percentage of body fat can be measured, ranging from measurement of skinfold thickness to ultrasonography. There are machines available on the market for laypersons to measure their own body fat percentage, but the most accurate measurements are performed in metabolic laboratories. If you would like to use any of the available tools to measure your body fat percentage, note that it is not as important to have the precise percentage but to use that number as a starting point upon which you would like to improve. For example, no matter what tool you choose to use, if your percent body fat comes up as 35 percent using the same tool you used to get that measurement, you can watch for any improvements relative to the baseline number.

Homework

Per the instructions above, determine your height, weight, and BMI. (Since many people overestimate their height, I recommend that you re-measure your height to ensure accuracy.) Measure your waist circumference. Record all of these values. Does your BMI accurately assess your overweight status? If so, set your goal for the BMI you would like to reach. Ideally, it will be below 25. Go back into the BMI calculator, and determine what you need to weigh in order for you to achieve a BMI of 24.9. That will be your initial target weight. You can adjust this number down if you wish once you achieve that target weight.

LABORATORY ASSESSMENTS FOR NUTRITIONAL HEALTH STATUS

· ·

Taking blood and urine samples are your physician's means to see if there are any signals to be concerned about with your health, with respect to nutritional status, diabetes, cardiovascular disease, and some cancers. Of course, this does not cover other necessary routine exams, such as mammograms, pap smears, prostate checks, and colonoscopies. These other screenings are outside the scope of this book. However, I highly encourage you to ensure you are receiving the right screening tests for your age and sex. Please discuss this with your physician. If the basic blood panels are normal, except in rare cases, it tells us that there is nothing further that needs to be tested at that time; you are fine. With a simple blood sample, the presence or risk of the chronic diseases in question is determined, as well as your nutritional status. The blood tests that should be ordered by your physician include a CBC (complete blood count), comprehensive metabolic panel, vitamin D level, thyroid panel, lipid profile, blood sugar (blood glucose) values both fasting and two hours after you have eaten (two hours postprandial), a C-reactive protein (CRP) level, and liver function tests. Depending on your age and personal or family history, your physician may also recommend you have an EKG (electrocardiogram) done. The urinalysis essentially tells your physician if your kidneys are spilling protein and/or glucose. It is abnormal to find either one in the urine. Also, if the urine is unusually dark, it may indicate you are not properly hydrated. Very dark urine sometimes indicates there is blood in it.

Note that I cannot provide exact laboratory values for normal ranges of the various blood tests discussed here, as those values differ from lab to lab. You will see what the normal ranges are for your laboratory on your lab results.

The CBC measures all of the blood cells (red and white blood cells), your hemoglobin and hematocrit, your platelets, and the size of your red blood cells. Among other things, your doctor can determine your immune status, how well your body is prepared to fight infections, or if you have an active infection. It can also signal if you are iron, vitamin B_{12}, or folic acid (another B vitamin) deficient. This test is particularly important for those following a vegan diet because without meat products or proper supplementation, they can become vitamin B_{12} and iron deficient. A B_{12} deficiency results in a type of anemia called pernicious or macrocytic anemia. To confirm the diagnosis, your doctor would likely order more blood tests.

If you do not take in enough iron, an iron deficiency anemia may exist. Your levels of hemoglobin and hematocrit would signal if you weren't getting enough iron. This is another potential deficiency in the vegan diet, so it needs to be properly supplemented. To confirm the diagnosis, your doctor will look for signs and symptoms you may have been having and may order a test for serum ferritin and transferrin. If you are iron deficient, your doctor will likely suggest you supplement with iron tablets, which is not a big deal for most people. Some people do experience significant constipation with iron supplements. You should discuss any untoward effects of any medicines or supplements with your physician.

The basic metabolic panel will signal any abnormalities in your electrolytes, your kidney function, your level of hydration, and your protein status. The level of serum creatinine in this panel may indicate that your kidney function (also called your renal function) is insufficient. This is one you should be particularly mindful about because unfortunately, there is more chronic kidney disease in patients than is being detected. A primary reason for this is because many physicians were taught to look primarily at serum creatinine level to detect problems with kidney function. If the serum creatinine appears normal or only slightly elevated, they may not look any further. However, estimated creatinine clearance provides a much more accurate picture of how the kidneys are functioning (also called eGFR or estimated glomerular filtration rate). There are different ways of calculating creatinine clearance, and all have their strengths and weaknesses. Some laboratories are now routinely reporting eGFR. If your doctor's laboratory is not reporting eGFR, then it is most prudent to ask your doctor what your creatinine clearance would be, based on your serum creatinine level. In practice most clinicians use the Cockgroft-Gault equation. You can find this calculation at http://www.globalrph.com/crcl.htm. Just enter your age, gender, height, weight, and serum creatinine level, and it will calculate your creatinine clearance for you. Anything less than 60 ml/min would be an alert for further evaluation. It indicates your kidneys are not filtering metabolites and toxins as well as they should be. This can result in various and serious health problems, such as electrolyte imbalances, cardiovascular disease, and severe anemia. Chronic kidney disease is most often caused by prolonged high blood pressure or poorly controlled diabetes.[4] And since your kidneys clear many medicines, if you have insufficient renal function, the dosages of your medicines may need to be adjusted downward for your safety.

I recently saw a woman in her late eighties who was 5'5" in height and weighed 60.8 kg (133.8 lb). Her serum creatinine looked normal at 0.9 mg/dl. However, upon calculating her creatinine clearance using the Cockcroft-Gault equation, she clearly had renal insufficiency at 38.2 ml/min. The dosages for many of her medications needed to be adjusted down for safety purposes. The comprehensive metabolic panel will also provide your albumin level, which is a good indicator of nutritional protein status. Protein is made up of building blocks called amino acids. Amino acids are needed for growth to repair body tissue and perform other bodily functions. There are many different types of amino acids, some of which our bodies can manufacture themselves. These are called nonessential amino acids. There are nine amino acids that our bodies cannot manufacture (called essential amino acids*) and must get from food sources. Many people are concerned that a vegan diet will not provide enough protein. This is a common misperception. While meat and dairy do provide good sources of protein, vegetable food sources can also provide enough essential amino acids to maintain health. You can prove this to yourself by visiting your doctor and having your blood drawn after following a vegan diet for a couple of months. If your albumin level is within the normal range, then you are getting enough essential amino acids, and have an adequate protein status. There is no evidence to the contrary on this subject, so don't be swayed by hucksters who say you need to supplement your amino acid intake with whatever protein supplement they are trying to sell to you.

On your basic metabolic panel, there will be a BUN level (Blood Urea Nitrogen). The BUN to serum creatinine ratio can alert your doctor in a number of ways. A normal BUN: creatinine ratio is 10–20:1 (ten to twenty times higher BUN than creatinine). If the ratio is higher, say 30:1, this may be indicative of dehydration or a more serious condition such as gastrointestinal bleeding. If there are no other symptoms of a more serious health issue, such as black tarry stools or other signs of gastrointestinal bleeding, then it is likely that you are just not drinking enough water. If the ratio is lower than 10:1 say 6:1, it is most

---

* The essential amino acids are histadine, isoleucine, leucine, lysine, methionine, phenylalanine, threonine, tryptophan, and valine.

likely due to problems with your kidneys; it helps confirm the diagnosis of renal insufficiency if your creatinine clearance was less than 60 ml/minute. The lower ratio can also be indicative of pregnancy, liver disease, or a diet too low in protein. In all cases, if the creatinine level is higher than normal and/or the creatinine clearance calculation is less than 60 ml/min, further investigation is warranted.

Vitamin D level has recently received much attention, mainly because of its association with osteoporosis and heart disease.[5,6,7] However, vitamin D deficiency has also been linked with complications in multiple sclerosis, type 1 diabetes, breast cancer, and others. Although our bodies can make vitamin D with enough sunlight exposure, most of us do not get enough sun exposure to prevent deficiency. And since the risks associated with sun exposure are well known, more sun exposure is not likely to be recommended by your doctor. Vitamin D is not easy to get through food intake; even foods that are fortified with vitamin D often will not provide enough vitamin D to prevent deficiency. Therefore, most of us need to supplement our vitamin D levels by taking a vitamin D supplement. Even if you are already taking a vitamin D supplement, it is a good idea to have your vitamin D level tested to make sure you are getting enough from your supplement. In my own personal experience, even though I was taking a multivitamin with vitamin D on top of one 400 IU capsule every day and a calcium supplement with vitamin D, my vitamin D level was on the low normal range. I started taking two capsules of the vitamin D supplement, and my levels are now midrange normal. If your levels are severely low, there are pharmaceutical mega supplements that your doctor may prescribe for you, up to the 50,000 IU range. It is an easy thing to fix if it is broken and can help save you from or help minimize the complications of vitamin D deficiency.

The thyroid panel is an important test to ensure your thyroid gland is functioning properly. Low thyroid levels can contribute to heart problems, as well as lowering your metabolism (causing you to be overweight) and raising your cholesterol levels, among other problems. High thyroid levels can predispose you to bone fractures and heart arrhythmias (irregular heart beat), among other problems. Problems with your thyroid can be effectively managed, but as with everything else, they first need to be identified.

The fasting lipid panel will indicate to you and your doctor if your cholesterol and triglyceride levels are too high, or in the case of HDL cholesterol, too low. LDL cholesterol is the bad cholesterol, responsible for building plaque in your cardiovascular system (called atherosclerosis), which is responsible for putting you at greater risk for heart attacks and strokes, as well as other circulatory problems. The HDL is the good cholesterol that helps to counteract what the LDL is doing. Thus, you want your LDL to be as low as possible and your HDL to be as high as possible. While lower is better with LDL, with no danger of ever being too low, there are recommended ranges established.[8, 9]

The levels of LDL cholesterol recommended are based on the number of risk factors you have for cardiovascular disease. The recommendations are based on sound evidence derived from analyzing many different scientific research studies. Risk factors include personal and family history, cigarette smoking, hypertension (high blood pressure), diabetes, male gender, advancing age, high saturated fat diet, HDL < 40mg/dl, and obesity. Your consumption of saturated fat, derived from meat products in the diet as well as trans fats, is the largest dietary contributor to your blood level of LDL cholesterol level. This may come as a surprise since most people believe that it is the cholesterol in the diet that causes their blood cholesterol to be elevated, but in fact, the greater contributor to blood cholesterol is the amount of saturated fat in the diet (see Table 1 for LDL level recommendations).

Table 1			
Risk Category	LDL Goal	Initiate Therapeutic Lifestyle Changes	Consider Drug Therapy
High Risk (10-year risk >20%)	<100mg/dl	≥100mg/dl	≥100mg/dl
Moderately High Risk (10-year risk10%-20%)	<130mg/dl	≥130mg/dl	≥130mg/dl
Moderate Risk (10-year risk<10%)	<130mg/dl	≥130mg/dl	≥160mg/dl
Lower Risk(10-year risk <10%, and 0-1 risk factors)	<160mg/dl	≥160mg/dl	≥190mg/dl
Adapted from The National Cholesterol Education Program Report: Implications of Recent Clinical Trials for the National Cholesterol Education Program Adult Treatment Panel III Guidelines. Endorsed by the National Heart, Lung, and Blood Pressure Institute, American College of Cardiology Foundation, and American Heart Association. Circulation, 2004; Vol. 110, pp. 227-239.			

Note that your risk category is determined by an equation that takes into account your age, gender, total cholesterol, HDL cholesterol, smoking status, systolic blood pressure, and if you are on medication to control your blood pressure. Your systolic blood pressure is the top number in your blood pressure reading. For example, if your blood pressure is 120/80, your systolic blood pressure is 120. The ten-year risk calculation is available at www. nhlbi.nih.gov/guidelines/cholesterol.

If you are unable to reach the target LDL levels through diet and weight loss, it is likely because you are genetically predisposed to having high LDL levels. Your liver just makes too much of it. In this case, you will need to take medications to reach the target. It is nothing to be ashamed of, and I recommend you don't fight it. It is of high importance to prevent heart attacks and strokes to correct the levels and keep them corrected. The drugs used to lower LDL cholesterol are very safe, with few side effects. Your doctor can monitor for these side effects.

The recommended HDL level is greater than 40 mg/dl, and greater is better, with no apparent limit. Lower levels put you at a higher risk for cardiovascular disease. HDL is not generally affected by your diet, but by your genetic propensity and level of exercise. If your HDL level is low, exercise can help raise the level. There are some medications that also raise HDL, but not by huge amounts, in general. Drinking red wine in moderation (we will discuss more about alcohol consumption later) can also help raise the HDL level. Discuss this with your physician to get his or her recommendation for a plan to raise your HDL level.

Very low density lipoprotein (VLDL) carries triglyceride throughout the bloodstream, so its level is strongly dependent on the triglyceride level. The target level for fasting triglycerides is less than 150 mg/dl. Higher levels predispose you to a greater risk for cardiovascular complications. High triglycerides can be due to being overweight, having poorly controlled diabetes, drinking too much alcohol, and/or eating too much sugar. They might also show as being high because you were not fasting for the blood test. You should be fasting for eight hours or longer before your lipid panel is drawn. In many cases, triglycerides can be controlled through weight loss, diet correction, and getting diabetes under control. If those efforts do not get them to the target level, there are medications that can help. Again, talk with your physician about his or her recommendations.

Blood sugar levels, both fasting (a minimum of eight hours not having eaten) and two hours after you have eaten (two hours postprandial) can detect diabetes and prediabetes (impaired glucose tolerance [IGT] and impaired fasting glucose [IFG]). Although many physicians still have their patients come in only for a fasting blood sugar, the two-hour postprandial level is oftentimes the first lab value to show that a person has prediabetes.[10] By the time the fasting blood sugar becomes diagnostic, the person may have already progressed to diabetes. Thus, I strongly encourage you to ask your healthcare provider to do both fasting and two hours after eating around 75–100 gm of carbohydrate (equivalent to 20 oz of orange juice, or your doctor may have you drink a sugar solution in the office). See Table 2 for blood glucose levels diagnostic for prediabetes and diabetes. If either of these levels is high, your physician may request an A1c be done. The A1c level reflects average blood glucose over the last two to three months, and is also diagnostic for diabetes.

Table 2		
Blood Test	Prediabetes	Diabetes
Fasting Blood Sugar	100-125mg/dl	>125 mg/dl
2 Hr. Postprandial Blood Sugar	140-199mg/dl	≥200mg/dl
A1c	5.7-6.4%	≥6.5%
Adapted from the American Diabetes Association's 2012 Position Statement of the Standards of Medical Care in Diabetes. Diabetes Care, Vol. 35, Supplement 1, Jan 2012, pp.S11-S63		

Remember that if you have prediabetes, there is hope in preventing type 2 diabetes. We will discuss this further in Part 4.

The C-reactive protein (CRP) level gives an indication of the level inflammatory response going on inside your body[11] and, if chronically elevated, can add to the predictive value of total and HDL cholesterol in determining the risk of heart attacks and strokes in both men and women.[12, 13] While there are also other biomarkers of inflammation, they are not yet routinely tested in practice. Be aware that recent trauma and infection can also cause the CRP level to become elevated. Thus, if your level is elevated, your doctor may wish to get a repeat blood sample at a later date to confirm the level is *chronically* elevated. There are a few means by which your CRP can be lowered. Following a vegan diet can actually reduce the level of CRP to the same extent as taking a statin![14, 15] Increasing physical activity can lower CRP level,[16] as can the statins used to lower LDL levels.[17] In fact, in a large study of over seventeen thousand healthy patients, rosuvastatin (Crestor®) was shown to reduce major cardiovascular events in apparently healthy persons without cholesterol problems.[18] It apparently did so by reducing the CRP levels on average by 37 percent. So even if your LDL level is good, if your CRP is chronically high, your doctor may recommend taking rosuvastatin to help bring the level down. You may wish to discuss with your physician your desire to try the 95% vegan approach first, given the data presented here. The key is that if you attempt to reduce the level with the 95% vegan approach, you need to recheck your CRP in about three months to ensure it has gotten your CRP level into the acceptable range. If not, it is time to seriously consider taking the statin.

Liver function tests (LFTs) can help detect numerous abnormalities, which can be due to a multitude of causes including liver damage from alcohol abuse, taking certain medications, viral and autoimmune hepatitis, gastrointestinal infection, and bile duct obstruction.[19]

To conclude, in a nutshell, unless you have some rare condition that dictates otherwise (and you would likely know this), the steps I have outlined for you in this chapter represent an excellent start to partner with your physician and monitor your own health and nutritional status. Since science is ever evolving, other measurements may make their way to the forefront for testing in your healthcare provider's office. If you stay current on scientifically validated instruments to test your health, you will remain effective at managing your own health with your healthcare provider.

Homework

If you have had recent blood work drawn at your doctor's office, request that a copy of your results be sent to you. Compare the results to the recommendations in this chapter. For each result, write down what the normal target range is for that value. Write down each result as indicated in Appendix 4, noting if it is normal, high, or low. That is the goal for which you will strive. If any levels concern you that have not already been discussed with your doctor, notify his or her office that you need to speak with your doctor. Ask for his or her recommendations, including when you should schedule your next appointment for follow-up.

If you have not had recent blood work drawn at your doctor's office, schedule an appointment for a routine physical. Then follow the instructions above. Also, be sure to drink plenty of water in the days before and on the day of having your blood drawn. Dehydration can skew blood test results and it is difficult to explain to a health insurance company that your tests might look sub-optimal because you were dehydrated. That said, if there is a problem with your blood tests, do not simply waive it off as dehydration without first discussing with your physician, since it *can* indicate a more serious problem. You can't fix something if you don't know it is broken. I implore you not to stick your head in the sand regarding your health; many health problems can be avoided or minimized through routine health checkups. Just feeling okay doesn't mean you are okay!

THE MACRONUTRIENTS, WATER, FIBER, ALCOHOL, AND ORGANIC

· ·

In this chapter, we will begin to get more specific about taking control of your dietary intake. Keep in mind that, although I will provide specific guidelines, if you are eating a vegan diet with a wide array of food choices, adding very little added fat, you will be getting what your body needs in terms of carbohydrate and protein.

The Macronutrients: Carbohydrate, Fat and Protein

Carbohydrate

Although demonized by fad diets, carbohydrate is essential for life.

> Myth: Carbs are bad for you.
>
> Fact: Regularly eating too much sugar, per se, is unhealthy, but healthy carbs are a necessary component of your diet.

It is the only form of energy utilized by the brain and is necessary to prevent an unhealthy rate of fat breakdown, which can lead to acidosis, a toxic condition that can damage your internal organs. Carbohydrate from whole food sources (vegetables, legumes, whole grains, and fruits) should represent the largest percentage of your overall caloric intake: 45–65 percent of your total calories, with no fewer than 130 grams per day.[1] To give you some idea of what this might look like from a dietary perspective, most vegetables contain around 5 grams of carbohydrate in one-half cup cooked. This includes vegetables such as broccoli, green beans, spinach, tomatoes, cauliflower, and collard greens. Starchy vegetables (examples include corn, green peas, lima beans, and baked beans) contain around 15 grams per one-half cup cooked. One slice of bread typically contains 15–20 grams of carbohydrate. One fruit serving (one small apple, fifteen grapes are examples of what one serving looks like) contains around 15 grams of carbohydrate. Pasta, noodles, and rice are also carbohydrate sources, with one half cup cooked containing around 15 grams.

A review of the scientific literature with respect to how well low-carbohydrate diets work reveals that the main reason for weight loss was that the diets had lower calorie intake and longer diet duration, not due to the reduced carbohydrate count.[2] This is identical to what we saw in our example gentleman in Part 1, Chapter 3. That being the case, does it make any sense to put yourself on such a restrictive diet, removing so many foods you love, when all you really need to do is lower your caloric intake overall? Not really. It makes far more sense, particularly in light of the data supporting a vegan diet to move toward 95% vegan, enjoying a wide variety of tasty dishes.

Carbohydrates are classified by how many sugar molecules are attached together. Monosaccharides have only one sugar molecule. Once eaten, monosaccharides absorb into the blood stream very quickly, generally raising blood sugar levels faster than more complicated sugars (there are some exceptions, such as fructose having a lower glycemic index than sucrose). Glucose is the standard for monosaccharides and is used to quickly raise blood sugar levels during episodes of hypoglycemia (low blood sugar) in people with diabetes. High fructose corn syrup can be made of different combinations of glucose and fructose, but they are each in their monosaccharide form.

Disaccharides contain two sugar molecules. There are many types, including sucrose (table sugar), which contains one molecule each of fructose (a monosaccharide) and glucose bound together. Lactose is also a disaccharide, containing one molecule each of galactose and glucose bound together. It is found in dairy products, such as milk and yogurt. Disaccharides are also absorbed into the bloodstream relatively quickly, rapidly raising blood sugar, though not quite as fast as glucose.

Polysaccharides are complex carbohydrates containing many molecules of monosaccharides linked together in different ways. Because of the different ways the monosaccharides are linked together, the polysaccharide may have completely different properties than the monosaccharide building blocks. Starches, flours, and cellulose are polysaccharides, as is pectin. Polysaccharides, which we will call complex carbs moving forward, are more slowly absorbed into the bloodstream. Thus, they generally do not cause a spike in blood glucose as do mono- and disaccharides. In fact, cellulose and pectin are forms of fiber, which are not absorbed into the bloodstream, and do not count toward the total carb intake. We will discuss more about fiber later.

There has been quite a bit of debate about the relevance of the glycemic index of various foods. The glycemic index is a standardized measurement comparing how foods increase blood sugar levels when compared to glucose or white bread. In order to know for sure what the glycemic index is for a food, biological experiments on humans must be performed. This is why there isn't an available glycemic index for every food out there.

Foods that rank higher on the glycemic index raise blood sugar levels faster and higher than foods that are lower on the glycemic index. Monosaccharides in general have the highest glycemic index, while polysaccharides have the lowest. Since most meals are a mixture of foods with different glycemic indexes, it is difficult, if not impossible, to forecast the glycemic index of a meal overall. Other dietary components, such as the fiber and fat in a meal, can influence the glycemic index of the entire meal. You can find a list of foods for which the glycemic index has been determined at http://www.health.harvard.edu/newsweek/Glycemic_index_and_glycemic_load_for_100_foods.htm.

While the glycemic index may be important, the American Diabetes Association statement on dietary carbohydrate intake[1] suggests that carbohydrate *load* is more relevant than glycemic index alone in predicting a meal's effect on blood sugar. Glycemic load is a calculation in which the glycemic index is multiplied by the total number of carbs, minus the grams of fiber, and divided by 100.[3]

$$\text{Glycemic Load} = \frac{\text{Glycemic Index} \times \text{Total Available Carbs}}{100}$$

Total Available Carbs = Total Grams of Carbohydrate - Grams of Fiber

A score of 1–10 is considered to be a low glycemic load, 11–19 is a medium load, and 20 or higher is considered a high glycemic load.

That makes sense. Both how fast and how much your blood sugar rises after eating carbohydrate-containing foods depends on *both* the glycemic index for a meal *and* the quantity of carb eaten. Another way to look at it is this: you can help prevent a high glycemic index food from spiking your blood sugar by not eating too much of it.

So why is it important to understand how to keep your blood sugar levels as even as possible? There are a couple of important reasons. First, high blood sugar stimulates the production and release of insulin. In people without diabetes, the amount of insulin secreted is in direct proportion to the amount and type of carbohydrate eaten. Insulin is an anabolic hormone, which means it can stimulate cell growth. It encourages the storage of fat, which we obviously want to avoid. A spike in insulin level can also cause a precipitous drop in blood sugar. This not only makes you feel bad, weak, and shaky; it secondarily causes a release of cortisol, epinephrine, growth hormone, and glucagon.[4] Although this is a natural protective mechanism to keep our blood sugar from going too low, it is a stress mechanism that has been implicated in cell aging, obesity, reduced immunity, insulin resistance, and cardiovascular disease.[5, 6] Also, prolonged increased insulin levels have been associated with colon, pancreatic, and breast cancer.[7, 8]

A rapid spike of insulin often makes you feel so weak and shaky that you overeat in the process of trying to make those symptoms go away. This of course can lead to overeating the number of calories you need, which then causes weight gain longer-term.

The bottom line is that we want to prevent spikes of insulin and avoid prolonged increases in insulin levels. Since we now know that the amount of carbohydrate consumed and the glycemic index are equally important, we need to focus on both. We need to balance the amount of simple sugars out by having a lower load of them (eating only small quantities at a time). This means that when you get that uncontrollable urge for your favorite candy bar, how about only eating a bite or two? It would lower the glycemic load. Thoroughly taste and enjoy each bite. The less you eat of it, the less your insulin level will spike. In other words, you need to learn to play the system so that you can enjoy some of these favorites from time to time, but do so in a way that does not cause a huge spike in insulin. Have a bite or two and put it down (or eat just one "fun size"). You can come back for another bite or two in an hour or two. Better yet, save it for another day. This way, your blood sugar is not peaking and crashing, causing you to feel so badly that you overeat to compensate. You are also not loading up in empty, nonnutrititive calories.

Complex carbs from whole grains and legumes generally do not create a spike in insulin level because the fiber in these foods slow the absorption of the carbohydrate into the blood stream, but again, this depends on the quantity eaten. So while we do want to increase our intake of these foods as 95% vegans, we still want to be aware of the quantity we are eating. Fat in the meal also slows down the absorption of carbohydrate into the blood stream, but we don't want to go an unhealthy route just to reduce the glycemic index.

How would you know if you consumed too much carbohydrate at a sitting? One telltale sign would be how you feel a few hours later, having not eaten anything since that last meal. While it may be normal to feel hungry, it is *not* normal to feel weak, shaky, and sweaty. These symptoms are good indicators that you are having either a low blood sugar or a precipitous drop in blood sugar following an insulin spike. Stop and think about what you ate and how much. The next time you consume a similar meal, cut down on the portion size and see if you can avoid the signs and symptoms of low blood sugar.

Refined carbohydrates, such as those contained in white flour, have been stripped of the whole grain, removing the most nutritious part of the food source. Refining also strips the food of fiber, which in part helps slow the absorption of the carbohydrate and prevent insulin spikes, when eaten with good portion control. It is best to steer clear of refined carbs, but when you do eat them, keep the amount you eat at a sitting to no more than 15–30 grams of carbohydrate to avoid an insulin surge.

Fruit juices, particularly some commercial brands that have added sugar, are similar to refined carbs, in that all of the fiber is removed. Commercially available fruit juice is oftentimes loaded with simple sugar, which can cause just as much of an insulin spike as a candy bar. This is why orange juice is recommended as a household item to treat hypoglycemia (low blood sugar) in people with diabetes who take certain medicines. Other than the juices you make yourself with your juicer, with few exceptions, it is best to steer clear of that aisle in the grocery store.

In terms of reading food labels to get some idea of the type of carb in it as well as glycemic load, note that carbohydrate is reported as follows:

Total Carb
Fiber
Sugars

The total amount of sugars equals the total amount of mono- and disaccharides. While fiber is technically a carbohydrate, since it is not absorbed into the blood stream, it doesn't count in the total carbohydrate. Also, if you subtract the total amount of sugars and fiber from the total carb, you will then know the total amount of complex carb (polysaccharides). For example:

Total Carb 20g
Fiber 1g
Sugars 12g

So for this food, there are 12 grams of sugar (equal to about 2–½ tsp. of table sugar), and 7 grams of complex carb (20 minus 7 minus 1 equals 12) in each portion size. Let's pretend that this particular food's label also tells us it has zero grams of fat and 2 grams of protein. We can surmise that the product would have a fairly high glycemic index because it is high in simple sugars, and contains a moderate amount of complex carb, with very little fiber and fat to counterbalance the glycemic effect. The point here is that you need to be aware of the amount of sugar in your foods in order to avoid having high blood sugar, then insulin spikes. The above example actually came from a commercially available soup. Let's compare that product to chickpeas (also called garbanzo beans):

Total Carb 20g
Fiber 7g
Sugars less than 1g

Although the total carb is exactly the same as the previous example, one portion size of these chickpeas has 7 grams of fiber, 2 grams of total fat (all unsaturated), and 6 grams of protein. Quite a difference from the commercially prepared soup, wouldn't you say? It has a very small amount of sugar, 7 grams of fiber, and 12 grams of complex carb. The fiber slows down the absorption of the carb, which helps prevent an insulin spike. This is one of the reasons why beans are such a good source of carbohydrate.

Although both products contain a total of 20 grams of carb, the chickpeas have a much lower glycemic load. Since they contain fiber that the soup doesn't have, the amount of available carb is less:

Chick peas: 20 grams total carb – 7 grams of fiber = 13
Soup: 20 grams total carb – 1 gram of fiber = 19

Right off the bat, there are clearly fewer available carbs in the chickpeas per portion size. Knowing that the fiber in the chickpeas will yield a lower glycemic index, you can reason that portion for portion, the chickpeas will not cause the insulin spike that the soup will cause. You don't necessarily need to actually calculate glycemic load to get a picture of which food is going to produce a higher surge of insulin, but it is good to know how in cases where it is not clear.

Let's examine how glycemic load may be impacting you via a Homework exercise so that you can compare a few different foods. Remember, the homework is there to help you solidify the learnings within that section, so please don't skip them.

Homework

Go to the Internet and open these two websites: http://www. health.harvard.edu/newsweek/Glycemic_index_and_glycemic_load_for_100_foods.htm, and www.calorieking.com. The first site is the Harvard Medical School list of glycemic index values for given foods. The second site will permit you to look up foods to find out how much total carbohydrate and total fiber is in each portion size so you can determine the total available carb: Total carb – Total fiber = Total available carb.

Grab three items you typically eat from your pantry, refrigerator, or freezer. On the Harvard site, look up what the glycemic index is per portion. Keep in mind the glycemic index does not change with varying portion sizes. It is always the same.

On the Calorie King site, search the food item, and be sure you enter the right amount for a typical portion size you would eat. Look at the carbohydrate amounts.

Fill in the following table to determine the glycemic load for each of your three items:

A	B	C	D	E	F	G	H
Food	Approximate Portion Size	Total Carb	Dietary Fiber	Available Carb (C - D)	Glycemic Index	Glycemic Load (E x F ÷100)	Low, Medium or High Glycemic Load?*
EXAMPLES							
Hummus	1/4 cup	8g	2g	6g	6	0.36	Low
Maple and brown sugar instant oatmeal	1 packet	33g	3g	30g	83	24.9	High
Pitted prunes	2 pitted	12g	1.5g	10.5g	29	3	Low
* 1-10 = low glycemic load, 11-19 = medium, 20 or greater - high glycemic load							

Now, think back to how any of these foods affected how you felt two to four hours after you ate them. Do you think they caused an insulin surge? If you cut your portion size in half, what would the glycemic load look like? Could you be making wiser choices with lower glycemic index choices? Now you are in control!

Fat

Ounce for ounce, gram for gram, fat supplies more than twice the calories of carbohydrate and protein. It has 9 calories per gram, versus 4 calories per gram for carbohydrate and protein. The real bad guy of the fat world is saturated fat. Most of the LDL (bad cholesterol) floating around in your blood vessels was made in your liver from saturated fat, not from dietary cholesterol. Non-vegans get most of their saturated fat from meat and dairy products. Both vegans and non-vegans get saturated fat if they choose food products containing hydrogenated oils, such as shortening and margarine, as well as some peanut butters. Just cutting out meat and dairy from your diet will markedly reduce the amount of saturated fat you are eating. However, some natural oils, such as coconut and palm oil, contain high quantities of saturated fat. The key to identifying saturated fat is how solid the product is at room temperature. For example, butter remains fairly firm at room temperature. Lard, fat extracted usually from beef, is even more solid at room temperature, indicating it is more saturated than butter. And although shortening is made strictly from vegetable oil, it is solid at room temperature due to the process of hydrogenation. This is a chemical process whereby unsaturated fats are converted to saturated fats by adding hydrogen. Partial hydrogenation simply means that not all of the fat in the product is hydrogenated.

It is also the process of hydrogenation that creates trans fats. Trans fats have recently received quite a bit of attention because of their disproportionate ability to influence risk factors that contribute to cardiovascular disease.[9] For example, just a 2 percent increase in caloric intake from trans fatty acids was associated with a 23 percent increase in cardiovascular disease! Since the FDA now requires food manufacturers to list the amount of trans fats on their food labels, it is easy to identify those products you want to avoid.

Monounsaturated fats are found in olive oil, canola oil, all of the nut oils (peanut, walnut, etc.), and avocado. They have been touted to help lower the risk of cardiovascular disease, and Americans have been adding it to their food with great vim and vigor, like sprinkles on an ice cream cone. But please allow me to set the record straight. The reason they appear to lower the risk of cardiovascular disease is because cultures that eat less saturated and trans fats and more monounsaturated fat (such as in the Mediterranean diet) tend to have lower rates of cardiovascular disease. The key here is that their diet *replaces* saturated and trans fats with monounsaturated fat; they do not just add it to their diet willy-nilly.

> Myth: Adding olive oil or other "healthy" oils on top of your diet is a healthy choice.
>
> Fact: Adding fat on top of your diet will not improve your cholesterol. Healthy fats are only beneficial if they replace less healthy fats, and either way you should strive to eat less fat overall.

We have missed the proverbial boat if we are adding monounsaturated fat to our diets and not replacing what we would normally eat in saturated fat. I have a friend who, for years, drenched her cooking in olive and peanut oils fervently insisting that they were good for her. For years, I told her that adding more fat to her diet was not good in any circumstance, particularly if she already had a cholesterol problem. Of course, she never had her lipid panel (cholesterol levels) drawn, so she really had no idea how adding all of the extra fat was affecting her health. Finally, she went for a routine physical during which her physician drew a lipid panel. Her LDL level was through the roof at around 185 mg/dl. No doubt the oils she was adding to her food were not helping the matter.

As a general statement for adults, you do not have to be concerned that you aren't getting enough fat. The Western diet supplies too much fat already. However, there are some essential fatty acids that you must get in your diet. Your body cannot manufacture them. Attention has recently been given to the potential for deficiency of omega-3 fatty acids, a type of essential fatty acid. The American diet, rich in omega-6 fatty acids, mostly from meat sources and oils, has caused concern due to the observations that tissue samples from Americans contain large amount of omega-6s and low levels of omega-3s, meaning our diet is disproportionately providing far more omega-6s than omega-3s, causing an imbalance. It has been observed that there tends to be abnormally low levels of omega-3s in people with certain diseases, such as cardiovascular disease, type 2 diabetes, rheumatoid arthritis, asthma, several cancers, and psychiatric disorders.

> Myth: You should get all the omega-6 and omega-3 fatty acids you can.
>
> Fact: While there is a minimum of each which comprise a healthy intake, the ratio of omega-6 to omega-3 fatty acids in your diet is important. You probably don't need to worry about omega-6s because our diets are fairly rich in them, so really focus on getting enough omega-3s.

Most foods high in omega-6 fatty acids are very low in omega-3 fatty acids. The Western diet indeed does have a relatively high ratio of omega-6 to omega-3 fatty acids, which appears to be part of the increase in inflammatory based diseases, such as those mentioned above. In that fish is higher in omega-3s, taking fish oil supplements helps to correct the imbalanced omega-6 and omega-3 ratio. Thus, fish oil supplementation became a standard recommendation to help prevent cardiovascular disease. As you will soon see, it is not necessary to use fish oil supplements to get your omega-3s.

A paper published in the *American Journal of Clinical Nutrition* was dedicated to attempting to set a standard for how much omega-3 was needed for optimal health.[10] As mentioned earlier, it appeared to be the ratio of omega-6 to omega-3 fatty acids that was the problem in the United States. Since different cultures consume different amounts of omega-6s, it is difficult to come up with a solid recommended daily intake of omega-3s to match the amount of omega-6 in each culture's diet to balance the amount of omega-6s eaten and cover all cultures in the United States and throughout the world. However, the paper did conclude that for an American diet containing 2,000 calories, approximately 3.5 grams of omega-3s is sufficient but much lower (down to one-tenth of that amount) would be sufficient if the diet was much lower in omega-6 fatty acids. To put this into perspective, one and a half teaspoons of flaxseed oil (a vegan product) contains about 3.5 grams of omega-3 fatty acids, which is plenty for most of the population. There are also flaxseed oil supplements on the market you can take if you are trying not to add any fat to your food. You can also substitute ground flaxseed (1 tbsp. + 3 tbsp. water) for each egg in a recipe to boost your omega-3 intake while lowering the amount of other fat and cholesterol you get from each egg. So as a 95% vegan you can use flaxseed instead of fish oil to obtain everything you need. Also, note that 3.5 grams of omega-3s in a 2,000-calorie diet is only 31.5 calories or 1.6 percent of the total daily caloric intake!

Having said all of the above, omega-6 fatty acids also contain essential fatty acids; the human body cannot manufacture them.

The American Heart Association has recommended that 5–10 percent of the total daily caloric intake consist of omega-6s.[11] For a 2,000-calorie diet, that would mean that 11–22 grams of omega-6 fatty acids would sufficiently cover this recommendation. Most vegans would not have to work to get enough omega-6s. For example, 1 oz of sesame seeds contains 6.7 grams of omega-6s. Soybeans contain 3.8 grams of omega-6s in just half a cup. The bottom line is that you really don't need to even think about whether you are getting enough omega-6 fatty acids.

To summarize, for a 2,000-calorie diet, one really only needs to get *at most* about 25–26 grams of fat per day: 3.5 grams of omega-3s and at most 22 grams of omega-6s. (For diets with lower amounts of calories, the amount of essential fatty acids needed would be proportionately lower.) Together, this represents at most 12 percent of the daily caloric intake as fat:

$$\frac{(3.5 \times 9) + (22 \times 9) \times 100}{2000} = 11.5\%$$

Considering the fact that the Western diet typically contains 40 percent or more of calories coming from fat, mostly omega-6s from meats and oils, you can easily see the concern about not getting enough omega-3s. You can also hopefully see that it is more prudent to worry about the following:

1. Getting too much fat than to worry that you aren't getting enough fat.

2. Whether you are getting enough omega-3 fatty acids in your diet versus the omega-6s.

3. Staying away from saturated fat as much as possible. For vegans, this means minimizing the amount of coconut and palm oils and hydrogenated oils.

4. Replacing the fat in your diet with omega-3 fats.

Now, let's boil this down to specific guidelines for *you*. This requires a Homework exercise.

Homework

Fill in the grid with your own information to get your specific healthy fat recommendations:

GUIDELINES FOR FAT INTAKE SPECIFIC TO YOU					
A	B	C	D	E	F
Desired Weight in Pounds*	Multiply desired weight in pounds by 15 for a quick approximation of calories per day to maintain that weight (Column A X 15)	Multply total calories by 1.6% (0.016) to get calories from Omega-3's (Column B X 0.016)	Divide total fat calories by 9 to get grams per day of Omega-3's (Column C/9)	Multiply total calories by 5% (0.050)) to get calories from Omega-6's (Column B X 0.050)	Divide by 9 to get grams per day of Omega-6's (Column E/9)
EXAMPLE:					
135	2025	32.4	3.6	101	11
*Refer back to the previous HOMEWORK assignment in which you identified the weight you need to be in order to have a BMI of less than 25. If BMI did not apply to you, then enter the weight you wish to maintain long-term.					

The purpose of this exercise is not to send you off in a wild frenzy of worrying if you are getting all of the perfect quantities of healthier fats. Rather, it is to draw your attention to just how little fat and what type of fat is required in our diets to maintain good health. In the example above, a person who wishes to maintain 135 pounds only needs about 3.6 grams of omega-3s and 11 grams of omega-6s. If this person were to cut out most of his or her omega-6s, even fewer omega-3s would be necessary to counterbalance. To put this into perspective, flaxseed oil contains approximately 55 percent omega-3s, 25 percent monounsaturated fatty acids, and 20 percent of omega-6s. Therefore, one teaspoonful of flax will yield about 3 grams of omega-3s, 1.25 gram of monounsaturated, and 1 gram of omega-6s. The bottom line is that since most food sources have a little bit of each type of healthy fat, eating a wide variety of whole foods as a 95% vegan and being a bit mindful about getting enough omega-3s should be just fine. It would not be helpful to go overboard on omega-3s. Remember, fat has 9 calories per gram. After you get what you need from the essential fatty acids, everything else is just calories potentially adding to your personal fat stores.

So the next time you are at a party and the conversation drifts to the concern that we have to make sure we are getting *enough* or the right type of fat in the diet (I have personally heard these conversations), you now have the scientific evidence to intelligently discuss a more appropriate viewpoint.

Protein

Protein is essential for tissue growth and repair, adequate immune status, and maintaining internal fluid balance. Although much attention is given to protein, mostly through commercials that are trying to convince the public that they need the supplement the company is selling, protein is sadly misunderstood. There are literally hundreds of scientific papers in the medical literature on the subject of protein needs. It is a complex subject in which much attention from global, credible, scientists has been given, so I urge you not to be led down the path of believing you need to buy protein supplements from a health food store salesperson.

In this section, we will boil down the credible volumes of science into prudent recommendations for you personally.

The truth is that we get far more protein in the Western diet than what we need. Although there is no evidence that this creates harm to those with normal kidney function, excess protein in the form of animal products is clearly associated with the diseases that are not seen as much in those who follow a vegan diet: obesity, type 2 diabetes, cardiovascular disease, and some forms of cancer. In addition, excess protein in the form of animal products inherently increases our intake of saturated fat. Even the leanest chicken contains three grams of fat per ounce!

Absolute protein requirements are most dependent on weight.[12] For women, 0.85 gram/kg (0.39 gm/lb) body weight is a good estimate. For men, around 1 gm/kg (0.45 gm/lb) body weight is a good estimate.[13] For women, as they get older, more protein may be needed to preserve muscle mass, ensure adequate calcium absorption, and help minimize bone loss—1 gm/kg (0.45gm/lb) body weight.[14, 15, 16] You may be interested to know that even in very sick patients in the hospital (cancer or burn victims), we usually provide 1.2 gm/kg (0.55gm/lb). We do not mega-dose even the sickest hospital patients with protein because it is not needed (tell that to the guy trying to sell you on the protein supplements). Of course, we ensure these patients get the right amount of carbohydrate and fat so that the protein is used to build healthy tissue and not used by the body as a calorie source.

Let's see what all of this means for you.

Homework

See the table below, and follow the instructions to get your personal protein requirement per day.

A	B	C	D	E	F
Gender	Age	Weight in Pounds	Divide Column C by 2.2 to get weight in kg	GM/KG Protein Required (1gm for men, 0.85gm for women under 65, and 1gm for women over 65)	Multiply Column D x Column E to get grams of protein required per Day
Male	18 and above			1.00	
Women	<65 years			0.85	
Women	≥ 65 years			1.00	
EXAMPLES					
Male	48	180	81.8	1.00	82
Female	36	135	61.4	0.85	52
Older Female	70	128	58.2	1.00	58

As you can see from the examples, a man weighing 180 pounds requires 82 grams of protein per day, a woman less than sixty-five years of age who weighs 135 pounds requires 52 grams of protein per day, and a woman over the age of sixty-five who weighs 128 pounds likely requires 58 grams of protein per day.

The average Western diet contains two to three times as much protein as is needed. It's no surprise that Americans are a stand-out population in terms of obesity and cardiovascular disease! Along with the excessive protein, we are getting far too much fat. By switching to vegetable sources for your protein needs, it is possible to cut out pretty much all fat. For example, legumes (beans and peas) and tofu contain very little fat. On the other hand, nuts and seeds contain quite a bit of fat. And just because nuts and seeds contain good fat, if you have a high LDL, no fat is a good fat for you, other than the bare essentials we discussed above. You would not be helping yourself to consume more nuts with the idea that they are heart healthy.

Now comes the question about the quality of protein in the vegan diet. Protein derived from animal sources has been tradi-tionally called *high biological value* or *complete protein* because it contains all of the essential amino acids* (the ones your body can-not manufacture). If you are getting all of your protein from plant sources, unless you get it all from isolated soy protein (you won't) or nutritional yeast flakes,** you will get more of certain essen-tial amino acids from beans and legumes and different essential amino acids from grains. And although it is still widely believed that because of the lower digestibility of plant foods versus ani-mal sources means vegans must eat more protein, studies show that there is not a significant difference in protein requirements based on the source of the protein intake.[17] This means that the amount you calculated for yourself above does not need to be

---

*   The essential amino acids are histadine, isoleucine, leucine, lysine, methionine, phenylalanine, threonine, tryptophan, and valine.

** Nutritional yeast flakes are used in many vegan recipes. Two table-spoons provides a whopping 8 grams of complete protein.

adjusted up because you will be getting the majority, if not all of your protein needs, from plant sources.

Beans and legumes are particularly high in lysine, while grains provide more methionine. Together, they provide complete protein. However, because your diet will be relatively high in grains (whole grain breads, rice, and pasta) already, you do not generally need to worry about whether you are getting enough methionine. Note also that all of the other essential amino acids pretty much balance out over your entire dietary intake.

Your attention should be more attuned to whether you are getting enough lysine than that of getting enough methionine. In addition to eating beans and legumes, you will get lysine through using soymilk, leafy green vegetables, potatoes (both sweet and white), and squash. Other vegetables also contain lysine, just in lesser quantities. This is why you always hear that with a varied diet; you can meet your nutritional needs.

Another theory we need to discuss is the one that tells us we must eat complementary proteins (meaning we need to complement foods high in one or more essential amino acids with other foods high in different essential amino acids in order to get complete protein) at the same time in order for the body to use the amino acid intake properly. This conventional wisdom has been disproven. Because muscles contain a pool of free amino acids for the body to use, particularly lysine, you do not have to ensure you eat complementary proteins within the same meal or even the same time span. In fact, as long as you average a sufficient intake of essential amino acids over several days, you should be fine.[18]

Up until now, there was no credible resource that outlined exactly how many servings of grains, legumes, and vegetables to eat daily to ensure you receive an adequate complementary protein intake for your given caloric needs. In this book's weight loss section, I will show you the recommended balance of legumes to grains for each calorie level you need to maintain an adequate protein intake. However, now that you know approximately how much protein your body requires on average, each day, you can compare the amount of protein you receive from different sources to your needs and estimate if you are getting enough overall protein. Through this strategy, then comparing to the recommendations I will provide you later in the book, and then seeing your blood work from your physician (albumin level, BUN:creatinine ratio), you will have an accurate picture of the adequacy of your dietary protein. If you feel good *and* your blood work looks good, you are doing a good job!

Finally, I would like to address the bad press soy has been getting lately about fear of increasing breast cancer risk. This is an important topic for your health knowledge if you are a woman. The fear of increased breast cancer risk comes from some of the data from animal studies and *in vitro* studies (test tube studies). The epidemiological studies in humans did not confirm what was produced in animal studies. However, as we discussed previously, it is very difficult to prove *cause and effect* for any single nutrient due to the many confounding factors in human nutritional research. The research on the relationship of soy to breast cancer is no exception; there are many conflicting study results out there. There are questions about whether the epidemiological results in one population of women are relevant to other populations of women. There are genetic differences, age differences, whether a woman is pre- or postmenopausal, how much soy they actually consumed, etc. As usual, there is no clear-cut answer, only a preponderance of the evidence that in humans, soy does not appear to increase the risk of a woman getting breast cancer.

Several patients have told me their physicians have advised them not to allow their daughters (childhood through adolescence) to consume products containing soy. This recommendation is based on the fact that the isoflavones in soy are chemically similar to estrogen. Since some breast tumors are estrogen-sensitive, they have rationalized that the isoflavones in soy can produce the same effects as estradiol, a stronger estrogen associated with breast cancer. This has not been demonstrated in human studies. To the contrary, it appears from epidemiological studies mostly conducted in Asian countries that soy consumption in younger years may actually be protective against breast cancer risk in later years.[19, 20, 21, 22, 23] Also in epidemiological studies, it appears that women who have had breast cancer and consume soy protein have lower rates of recurrence than women who do not.[24] A theory behind why soy *may* be protective against breast cancer is that isoflavones have anti-estrogen properties by blocking the more potent forms of estrogen from binding to the estrogen receptors in the cancer cells. It is like placing a key into a lock. No other key can go in the lock as long as that first key is in there. In other words, as long as the weaker estrogens in isoflavones are bound to the estrogen receptor, the more carcinogenic estrogens cannot bind to the receptor.

Soy opponents will argue that there is very little evidence in controlled clinical trials to prove what has been observed in the epidemiological studies. That is fair push back, based on what we discussed in Part 1 with respect to nutritional health claims. However, there are also no controlled studies that demonstrate soy has a role in *causing* breast cancer. The worst-case scenario appears to be that soy may not be protective in *preventing* breast cancer. The quantity of soy consumed by women in Asian countries does appear to reduce breast cancer risk, but again, there are so many other variables to consider: their levels of exercise, tea and other antioxidant intake, low animal product consumption, etc. So while we might be able to say there is a *correlation* between soy intake and a reduced risk of breast cancer, we cannot say there is *cause and effect* between increasing soy intake and reducing breast cancer risk. This is an important distinction.

Given the entire body of literature on the subject, I will place my bet on soy being a good source of protein to replace animal protein. It is not my only source of protein, but I don't intentionally minimize my intake for fear it will cause breast cancer either.

Although we will discuss organic products later in the book, let me also state here that I do recommend eating only organic soy products, particularly if you are in any way concerned about soy and breast cancer. We do not yet know the full potential effects of GMOs, so I recommend you stay away from them.

Having said all that, I also want you to be aware that there is no evidence that taking isoflavone *supplements* will produce the same protective effect that soy-containing *foods* do. There is also no proof that supplementing the diet with more isoflavones than what is present in food is safe or effective. Foods containing soy also have other protective effects beyond the isoflavones, which these supplements do not mimic. So once again, I recommend you avoid the temptation to buy into what the supplement sales-person tells you and replace some of the protein you used to get from meat with more soy products.

WATER

· ·

Water is the most important nutrient of all, in that we cannot live without it for as long as we could other nutrients. It comprises approximately 75 percent of muscle mass, and only 10 percent of fat mass. Since men generally have a higher muscle mass than women, their body composition is much higher in water. For all of us, water makes up anywhere from 60–75 percent of our entire bodies!

Water enables our organs to function properly by helping to flush out toxins. We need it for our bodies to make new blood cells and plasma (the liquid that blood cells float around in). Depending on your age, health status, climate in which you live, amount of exercise and gender, your need for water can be anywhere from eight 8 oz glasses of fluid per day to thirteen 8 oz glasses per day. All fluid and beverages consumed count toward this total needed per day. Frozen desserts such as sherbet, soups, and puddings also count toward fluid requirement. If you have normal kidney function, you can gauge your level of hydration at home by how often you have to urinate and the color of the urine. The less frequently you urinate and the darker the color of urine, the more dehydrated you are. Keep in mind, though, that it is also not necessarily safe to drink so much water that your urine has almost no color. As I mentioned in Part 2, the comprehensive metabolic panel drawn at your doctor's office or lab can also indicate if you are dehydrated.

How long could you live without water? It depends. While someone lost in the woods in a cool climate might live for a week without water, a baby left in a hot car can dehydrate and die in minutes.

Have you ever thought about the quality of the water your drink? This is something I am advising you to think about, investigate, and, if necessary, take steps to improve. If your water supply comes from a city waterworks, it must meet the minimum Environmental Protection Agency (EPA) standards for potential contaminants, such as microorganisms, volatile organic chemicals, and inorganic chemicals such as lead, mercury, chromium, etc. (see http://water.epa.gov/drink/standardsriskmanagement. cfm). Your city can set its own standards for water quality, which can be more stringent than the EPA guidelines, but never less stringent than EPA guidelines. If your water supply comes from a well, you are pretty much on your own to ensure your water is safe to drink and bathe in.

There are all sorts of potential water contaminants out there, including pesticides, disinfectants, radioactive substances, and dangerous byproducts of industry, such as chromium VI (also called hexavalent chromium). The good news is that the EPA and cities are on top of water testing and have maximum levels allowed where there is science to support maximum safe levels. The bad news is that science is ever evolving, and what was considered safe ten years ago may not be considered safe today. Thus, we may have been exposed to toxic levels of various chemicals through no fault of the EPA—the science may just not have been there at the time. The other bad news is that if there is a water main break, your water can become easily contaminated to the point where it is considered not potable (not safe to drink) or even safe to bathe in. Again, if you are on well water, it is up to you to ensure your water is safe. Let's discuss this further.

NSF International (National Sanitation Foundation), a not-for-profit, nongovernmental organization, is the leading global provider of safety standards for concerned citizens worldwide. It certifies various products through testing and retesting to meet their set standards, including drinking water purification systems. You can find the standards for drinking water at http://www.nsf.org/business/drinking_water_treatment/standards.asp. There are three standards to be aware of in terms of removing contaminants from drinking water:

1. NSF 42—A filtration system meeting this standard improves the aesthetics of the water. It reduces odors, removes particulates, and reduces chlorine. Many refrigerators with water dispensers have this level of filter.

2. NSF 53—A filtration system meeting this standard reduces specific contaminants that can affect health, such as lead and volatile organic chemicals (VOCs) such as benzene, and microorganisms such as Cryptosporidium and Giardia. It filters out chemicals that have a molecular weight or atomic mass roughly of one hundred or more. The terms molecular weight and atomic mass refer to the size of the contaminant. Lead has an atomic mass of around 207, so a product that meets NSF 53 would filter it out.

3. NSF 58—A filtration system meeting this standard cleans water through a reverse osmosis system, which further reduces contamination from additional potential poisons such as trivalent and hexavalent chromium (chromium III and chromium VI respectively), nitrates, and other dissolved solvents. It also removes fluoride and other minerals. Essentially, it removes smaller molecules than filters satisfying NSF 53, less than 100 molecular weight or atomic mass. The atomic mass of hexavalent chromium VI is 43, much smaller than lead. Flouride's mass is around 18.

The NSF standard to cover softening hard water, particularly for those on well water is NSF 44. Other NSF standards cover different methods of purifying drinking water (mostly for public waterworks), and filter systems for shower and bath.

There are many good filtration systems on the market that meet NSF 42 and 53 standards. You can choose whether you would want an above-the-counter model, which attaches directly to your sink faucet, or an under-the-counter system, in which another hole is drilled for an additional faucet. If you already have a filtration system or are using a product that is a pitcher with a filtration system, you may want to do a little digging to determine which NSF standards the product meets. Most of the pitcher-type models only cover NSF 42, however some do cover NSF 53.

Reverse osmosis systems satisfying NSF 58 are also available for residential use. Many of these systems require an under-the-counter configuration, in which you would gain an additional faucet. However, above-the-counter models are now emerging. The price of these systems has come down tremendously very recently, and so are affordable for much of the population. If you are handy as a plumber, you can probably install the system without any help.

If you have ever seen the movie *Erin Brockovich*, you know it was based on a true story about a lawsuit against PG&E (Pacific Gas and Electric) for contaminating a wide stretch of land in Hinkley, in the Mojave Desert in California with chromium VI. The chromium VI, used as an anticorrosive agent for their cooling towers, found its way into the water supply of Hinkley, resulting in numerous health problems for its residents, including cancers and aborted pregnancies. While chromium III occurs naturally on earth and is good for the body if not overdosed, chromium VI is a manmade form of chromium. It infiltrates our water system from industrial waste. There is nothing good about chromium VI; it is poisonous. Sadly, PG&E actually tried to convince the residents of Hinkley that the chromium contamination was actually good for their health.

Chromium III can convert to chromium VI through oxidation, and chromium VI can convert to chromium III through reduction. Reduction is accomplished by putting a chemical in an acidic environment. A good way to think of this is if you think of a sliced apple. If you leave it open to air, it will become oxidized and turn brown. However, if you sprinkle the apple with lemon juice, which is acidic, it protects against oxidation through reduction, and the apple does not turn brown. How this applies here is that even if you ingest chromium VI, the acid in your stomach can reduce some of it into chromium III if you are in reasonably good health (i.e., your gastrointestinal tract is intact). People who have compromised health, such as cancer and HIV patients, may not have the full function to reduce chromium VI into chromium III.

Personally, I do not feel the need to have a reverse osmosis system to remove chromium VI from my water supply due to the following: there is some evidence that in healthy people, concentrations of chromium VI of up to 2 mg per liter (2mg/L) are quickly reduced in the stomach to chromium III and thus should not produce health issues.[25] This would be like having a single grain of salt in a quart of water. While this seems reassuring, if your water is contaminated with high levels of chromium VI, it would overwhelm your stomach's capability to convert it to chromium III. You would also absorb some through your skin, as well as inhale some while in the shower, giving you an even higher level of exposure. Inhaled chromium VI is a known and potent carcinogen. This is no surprise, in that inhaled chromium VI doesn't come in contact with stomach acid that could reduce chromium VI to chromium III. The EPA standard calls for public drinking water to be at or below 100 parts per billion, which equates to 0.1mg per liter (0.1mg/L), which equals 100 micrograms/L. Since chromium testing includes all forms of chromium, for safety, the EPA assumes that *all* of the chromium level in a water sample is 100 percent chromium VI. The EPA's recommendations are continuously updated as new science provides additional information. The concentration of chromium VI of Hinkley's water was 0.58 ppm, or 0.58 mg/L, which equals 580 micrograms/L, almost six times the level considered safe by the EPA.[26]

In my city, Atlanta, the city watershed has set the chromium VI standard at 0.016 mg/L, or 16 micrograms/L, well below the safe limit established by the EPA. In looking at my city's water inspection report, there does not seem to be any chromium VI in our water supply. Thus, I do not feel the need to invest in a reverse osmosis system for my home. If I was immunocompromised from radiation, chemotherapy, or other condition, or I was on well water, I would likely view it differently.

Chromium VI is a good example to illustrate the workings of federal, state, and local governments with respect to ensuring the safety of our public water supply. However, it is just one example of a toxic substance. Many others exist.

Frankly, I worry more about the medications people flush down the toilet than I do chromium VI. Fortunately, the molecular weight of most drugs is greater than 100, so would be filtered out with my filter that satisfies NSF 53. For example, estradiol, a potent estrogen implicated in breast cancer, has a molecular weight of 272. Thus, NSF 53 certified filtration systems should have no trouble filtering it out of our drinking water. In that there are mutations occurring in wild fishes related to estradiol contamination, such as males having early stage eggs in their testes,[27] I don't think it is a huge leap to reason that people too may be having health consequences from inadvertent exposure to estradiol. And this is only one drug; there are thousands more we could be being exposed to. There are no EPA guidelines covering drugs as contaminants as of the writing of this book. And while it may be that the purification systems used by the public waterworks may reduce or eliminate drugs and their byproducts in our water supply, because they are not testing for drugs, we really don't know whether our water is contaminated with them or not. I recommend we all err on the side of safety and install, at a minimum, an NSF 53 certified filtration system. For further reading on this subject, please visit http://www.poison.org/current/water%20supply.htm.

The decision of whether or not to buy a filtration system for your water supply and what NSF standards you would want your filtration system to meet is completely up to you. You can test your water supply yourself for all sorts of chemicals. What you need to be aware of is at what level of the chemical the test would indicate a positive result that it is indeed in your water supply

Unfortunately, some of the tests are not very sensitive—that is, they do not detect the substance at a low enough level. For example, most of the available chromium VI tests only detect it at a concentration of 0.2 mg/L, which is twice as high as the EPA standard. There are more sensitive tests, but they come at a considerably higher price.

There are a variety of ways to determine the safety of your water supply. This requires a Homework exercise.

Homework

1. Whether you are on city or well water, get the list of the national drinking water standards from http://water.epa.gov/drink/contaminants/upload/mcl-2.pdf.

2. If you are on city water, you can go to http://cfpub.epa.gov/safewater/ccr/index.cfm?Open View to view the most recent water testing report for your water provider. Compare it to the drinking water standards.

3. If you are on well water and do not routinely monitor your water supply, you can request an agent test a sample for

known poisons (on the list you obtained from step 1). Go to http://www.cdc.gov/healthywater/drinking/private/wells/faq.html to find out how to get your water tested. As you will see, the EPA clearly states that you are responsible for the safety of your own well water. Click on all of the applicable links to thoroughly learn what you do not yet know. You can either have your water tested for you through a company (or sending in a sample to a laboratory) or you can purchase a testing kit and do it yourself. Please be aware that many at-home testing kits may only test for hardness, chlorine, and microorganisms. You want more thorough testing than that. Just be sure you know what you are getting before you invest.

4. Based on what you have learned about your drinking water, decide whether or not you believe you need a filtration or reverse osmosis system. The decision is entirely up to you.

5. Once you decide if you need a system and desired NSF standards it will need to meet, you can either shop locally for it or Google for "water purification systems." You will find a multitude of choices out there.

FIBER

• •

There are two classifications of fiber: soluble and insoluble. Soluble fiber becomes somewhat gelatinous in the GI (gastrointestinal) tract. To some extent, it adsorbs cholesterol and saturated fat, preventing them from being absorbed into the blood stream. Good sources of soluble fiber are beans and legumes, oats, psyllium, and flaxseeds. Insoluble fiber remains pretty much intact throughout the GI tract. Insoluble fiber is what we typically refer to as roughage. It is the most helpful in providing bulk to help reduce constipation. Good sources of insoluble fiber include whole grains, bran, and vegetables. Most foods that naturally contain fiber are a mixture of both but are classified by which type they contain more of. Recommendations for fiber intake are for total fiber and do not delineate between soluble and insoluble. They each have a role for good health.

The topic of fiber in our diets has been exhaustively discussed in the public arena, including:

1. The relationship between fiber and obesity, the more fiber that is eaten in a given population of people, the lower the rate of obesity, [28]

2. Its ability to help control diabetes, [29]

3. The belief in its potential to reduce the risk of colorectal cancer (Although in a large pooled analysis, when other

dietary factors were adjusted for, fiber was not shown to prevent colorectal cancer[30]), and

4. Its positive effects on blood pressure and cholesterol levels. [29, 31]

Other protective effects of fiber have been studied but have not borne out in controlled clinical studies. However, since populations with high fiber intakes do typically have lower rates of all of the above, for healthy adults, it is prudent to ensure your dietary intake of fiber is as high as possible.

The recommended amount of total fiber in the diet for normal, healthy adults is 14 grams per 1,000 calories, roughly 25 grams per day for women, and 38 grams per day in men.[32] Most people who eat a Westernized diet don't come close to having that amount. My personal opinion is that Westerners simply aren't hungry for healthy fruits and vegetables because they are so satiated—that is, they feel full and satisfied—by meat and dairy products, including fast foods. Once you begin your journey to veganism, you will quickly see that you are hungry for and will eat more vegetables, fruits, legumes, and whole grains. As a precautionary note, if you do not consume enough liquid in your diet and/or do not do any form of exercise, you are likely to become very constipated. If you do become constipated, a stool-softening laxative (such as Colace®, which is docusate sodium) with plenty of water is a good first option to overcome it. If this doesn't help, and you have normal kidney function, you can use a saline laxative such as milk of magnesia or magnesium citrate (also called citrate of magnesia), along with drinking more fluid. Stimulant laxatives such as those containing senna or bisacodyl can be used as either an oral formulation or as a rectal suppository. I only recommend you use these if either the above doesn't work or if you cannot take magnesium-containing products. Taking stimulant laxatives for more than a few days can cause your GI tract to slow down to the point where you can't defecate without them, so only use them sparingly, if at all. If you experience abdominal pain, you need to see your doctor.

Let's take a look at how simple it will be for you to get enough fiber in your diet as a 95% vegan. This requires a Homework exercise:

Homework

1. Once again, let's open www.calorieking.com. You can use any other resource at your disposal instead, if you wish.

2. Please look up the amount of fiber in one half cup white beans, one cup cooked broccoli, one half cup texturized vegetable protein (TVP which you will use as a ground beef replacement), a 2 oz serving of Barilla® whole grain spaghetti, one cup fresh strawberries, and one medium-sized sweet potato. Add up the total amount of fiber in all of these products. Did you discover that these foods would meet your daily fiber needs? See the next page for the answer.

Answer to homework on fiber quantities: The total amount of fiber for all of the foods listed is 31.3 grams. Consider that this does not even constitute a whole day's meals for a man or a woman!

ALCOHOL

Whether or not you choose to drink alcohol in any form is a choice only you can make. It does have its benefits and risks.

If you do drink alcohol, be aware that both the American Heart Association and the American Cancer Society recommend no more than one drink per day for women and no more than two drinks per day for men.[33, 34] One drink is equal to 12 ounces of beer, 5 ounces of wine, or 1.5 ounces of 80 proof distilled spirits. Higher consumptions than the maximum recommendations have been associated with an increased risk of developing breast cancer, cancers of the mouth, larynx, and esophagus; and cardiovascular disease. For people who are at risk for developing dependence, it is best to abstain from alcohol completely. Women who are pregnant or planning to become pregnant should also abstain completely.

We need to understand that these recommendations come from the totality of all of the available scientific data; these are the most rationally concluded recommendations. For example, while there is some evidence that the consumption of up to two drinks per day, three or four times per week may reduce the risk of heart attacks, higher levels of drinking appear to increase the risk of hypertension, which is a risk for heart attacks. If you do not drink, it is not recommended that you start. The evidence is not sufficient to support the recommendation that you start drinking. If you drink, even within guidelines, take precautions not to drive or operate heavy machinery.

I am often asked about red wine as a potentially better source of alcohol due to the apparent advantages of the polyphenolic compounds in red wine, such as flavonoids and resveratrol. In fact, scientific studies do support these compounds as being protective in the start and progression of atherosclerosis. Coupled with the fact that all alcohol in the recommended maximum quantities can elevate your HDL (the good cholesterol), I have to agree that choosing red wine over other alcoholic options appears to be the better choice.[35] Keep in mind that alcohol contains seven calories per gram, all empty calories when consumed in excess of the maximum recommended for health.

This section would not be complete without addressing the increasing problem of binge drinking. More than 38 million US adults binge drink about four times a month. Binge drinking is defined as a man consuming five or more drinks or a woman consuming four or more drinks within about 2 hours.[36] Binge drinking is responsible for many dangerous behaviors that result in car and other heavy machinery accidents, suicides, violence, and contracting HIV and other sexually transmitted diseases. All of this is very costly, both in dollars and in human lives. For more information, please visit http://www.cdc.gov/vitalsigns/bingedrinking/

ORGANIC OR NOT?

· ·

When it comes to whether organically grown food is more nutritious and safer, everyone seems to have an opinion. Here we will look at the currently available evidence.

In the United States, the US Department of Agriculture (USDA) defines the term "organic." Organic essentially means that the food was grown without unapproved chemical pesticides, herbicides, hormones, genetic modifications (no GMOs), and has not been irradiated. Note that there *are* approved methods for organic farmers to control diseases and pests in their crops. For example, the antibiotics streptomycin and tetracycline are approved for use to control a bacterial disease called fire blight in apples and pears. For the list of approved substances, see http://www.ams.usda.gov/AMSv1.0/getfile?dDocName=STEL PRDC5068682.

The definition and regulations for organic farming can be found at http://www.ams.usda.gov/AMSv1.0/nop. Foods cannot be legally labeled as being organic unless they were grown in accordance with the USDA standards.

Foods that are not organically grown are treated with a number of different chemical pesticides and herbicides. To monitor these chemical's potential effects on health, in 1993 the National Institutes of Health, including the National Cancer Institute, the National Institute of Environmental Health Sciences, and the EPA, began a study called The Agricultural Health Study.[1] It was a preplanned (prospective) study conducted in Iowa and North

Carolina intended to follow the disease risk (cancer and non-cancer) following the exposure to over fifty different pesticides. The study is still ongoing and includes eighty-nine thousand participant farmers as well as their spouses and children. The farmers, their spouses, and children who helped on the farm as pesticide applicators are routinely exposed to pesticides through their work. However, even spouses and children who did not directly apply pesticides are exposed to the pesticides environmentally, as well as through clothing with pesticides that were washed with the applicator's clothing. The level of exposure is determined both by responses to questionnaires and as well as through the collection of biological samples (urine and mouth cells).

Updates to the data collected in the study have been published frequently (see http://aghealth.nci.nih.gov/results.html#facts for specifics). Substudies to evaluate risks of various diseases have been conducted and published. As of this writing, in general, pesticide applicators and their families appear to have a 60 percent lower rate of death due to cardiovascular disease, diabetes, COPD, and total cancer than non-applicators in these states, which may be related to their lower tobacco use and greater physical activity. However, there are some concerning trends regarding specific cancers and other diseases.

There appears to be a two-fold increased risk for Parkinson's disease in applicators versus non-applicators. Male farmers who are applicators have a greater incidence of prostate cancer, and female farmers and spouses of farmers have an increased incidence of melanoma, breast, and ovarian cancer. Other cancers seen more frequently include lung, colon, and blood-related cancers. And although *cause and effect* have not yet been established, there does appear to be a *correlation*. The researchers hope to isolate the cause(s) of the increased incidence of these cancers in the coming years. Retinal degeneration, the leading cause of visual impairment in adults, appears to be associated with applicators reporting higher exposure to fungicides. And while certain pesti-

THE 95% VEGAN DIET

cides appear more likely to be responsible for the various health outcomes than others, I think we do have to acknowledge the fact that the study is ongoing and more data will come. Additional pesticides may crop up as a risk for disease but may just have a more latent effect (meaning that it may just take more time for these effects to be seen).

The results of the Agricultural Health Study are concerning. And while we are reminded these results of the study should be tempered by remembering that the study is being conducted in people who have a much higher acute exposure to these chemicals than the average person (including the fact that some of these people were involved in spills that were not promptly cleaned up), we must also consider how long these chemicals remain in the soil and how they spread to other areas. In fact, in a recent paper published in the *Annals of Internal Medicine*,[2] in which a systematic review of the literature from 1966 through May 2011 was conducted, approximately 70 percent of *organically* grown food had detectable levels of pesticides. This speaks loudly of the level of contamination in our soil of existing and previously used pesticides since they are not permitted for use in growing organic crops.

The overall conclusion of the *Annals* paper is that there is no overwhelmingly strong evidence that organically grown food is superior to conventional food from a *nutritional* standpoint. However, while there may not be strong evidence demonstrating superiority of the *nutrient* content of organically grown food, the authors still had to concede that by consuming organic food, we would reduce our exposure to *pesticides*. While this study was widely publicized to minimize the benefits of organically grown food, in my opinion, the importance of the potentially increased safety from reduced exposure to pesticides and herbicides was underappreciated. For example, let's consider an old nemesis banned in the 1970s: DDT. DDT is an organochlorine and was a commonly used pesticide until it was banned in 1972. It was initially used in World War II to control malaria, typhus, body lice, and bubonic plague.[3] It was inexpensive, effective, and lasted long in the environment, all of which appeared to be benefits. Then came the toxic effects in the environment. Wild birds and fish became highly affected. The birds began having reproductive problems, and offspring born had increased mortality rates. Fish were dying from DDTs toxic effects. It was then discovered that it deposited into the fat reserves of mammals, including humans. When fat breaks down, the DDT is released into the bloodstream, even finding its way into breast milk. DDT was ultimately banned as a probable carcinogen because of the effects on wildlife, but it was never proved to be a carcinogen in humans. That doesn't mean DDT isn't a carcinogen or isn't toxic to humans; it means there were inadequate data to prove it so. In fact, DDT stored in the fat of humans is mobilized during pregnancy and lactation, potentially affecting generations of people. It is good that DDT was banned when it was, but the problem is how long the chemical persists in our environment. In soil, DDT has a half-life of fifteen years. In groundwater, the half-life can be as long as thirty-one years. To put this into perspective, it takes five to seven half-lives for a chemical to be considered eradicated from its source. Thus, DDT is still found in our environment in appreciable quantities forty years after it was banned! And since there are not any ongoing studies specifically looking at the effects of DDT in humans, we may never fully understand how it has impacted our children and us. I use the example of DDT to illustrate the fact that while fifty or more different pesticides are being investigated in the Agricultural Health Study, we may not know the full extent of their impact on our health for decades to come and in fact may never know if it is not actively studied, as in the case with DDT.

None of the studies in the systematic review published in the *Annals* paper about organic food specifically addressed genetically modified (also called genetically engineered or bioengineered) food. This is a hotly contested, politically charged subject. Many crops have been genetically modified since 1996 in the United States, particularly corn, soy, potatoes, tomatoes, and canola. They are generally modified to be more resistant to insects, herbicides, and for improved growth. However, in some cases, genetic modification can also change the nutritional value of the food. For example, if genetic traits of corn are inserted into canola, it can change the fatty acid content from having a high content of omega-3 fatty acids to polyunsaturated fatty acids. On the other hand, it is also possible to improve the nutritional content through genetic modification. The problem is, you don't really know what you are eating if the food labels are not clear. Since these products are then sold to food manufacturers as ingredients, they then find their way into processed foods. Therefore, we can easily surmise that most US citizens eat genetically modified food on a regular basis without knowing it. Note that there is no law requiring food companies to include the fact that the ingredients in a processed food item contain genetically modified organisms (GMOs). In fact, the FDA only requires that genetically modified food be "substantially equivalent" to the naturally grown food product.[4] If the *overall* macronutrients of the item in question resemble that of the organically grown product and the item does not contain immediately identifiable toxic substances, the FDA will consider that item to be substantially equivalent. However, considering that genetically modified food only became widely used in the mid-nineties, and often in our history, there have been health consequences of man-made products identified decades after their widespread use; we may not yet be able to appreciate the health consequences of genetically modified foods in humans. In contrast, consider immediately recognized problems, such as salmonella outbreaks, which can quickly be associated with eating foods contaminated with it. Genetic modification of foods would not likely cause such an immediate health concern, other than acute allergic reactions to foreign proteins that were expressed from the genetic modification. Carcinogenic substances throughout our history have only been identified after years of exposure and subsequent cancer cases arising.

An interesting dichotomy exists between the American Medical Association (AMA) and the American Academy of Environmental Medicine on the subject of the safety of genetically modified foods. The AMA's executive summary regarding the safety of bioengineered food products states that "Bioengineered foods have been consumed for close to 20 years, and during that time, no overt consequences on human health have been reported and/or substantiated in the peer-reviewed literature."[5] On the other hand, the American Academy of Environmental Medicine (AAEM) cites recent studies demonstrating health effects of genetically modified foods on animal models, including infertility, internal organ damage, and immune dysregulation.[6]

So the bottom line of where we are with respect to fully understanding the potential long-term health consequences of genetically engineered food products in humans is that the jury is still out. Both the AMA and AAEM are correct. And it is true that the FDA's labeling requirements are lax. It is completely voluntary for food companies to label their products genetically engineered, however companies that use non-GMO options will proudly display it on their labels. Personally, I have not read any food labels that disclose the use of genetically modified ingredients in the manufacturing process, and don't anticipate I will see any food labeled that way unless it is mandatory.

This is a situation where we must make our own choices, based on who we choose to believe, while additional scientific evidence proving or disproving adverse health effects evolves. The only way to ensure we are not eating genetically modified food is to buy organic.

So there are three main issues to consider when it comes to choosing to buy organic food or not:

1. Is it better nutritionally? The answer to that question at this point in time appears to be no.

2. Is it safer? For pesticide exposure, the answer is yes. For genetically engineered food, the answer is maybe. (Keep in mind that we are still in the infancy stage in terms of gathering scientific information of the health effects of genetically modified foods.)

3. Is it affordable? Only you can decide that.

Now let's think of the bigger picture. If we all keep buying foods containing high levels of pesticides and foods that have been genetically modified, what is the incentive for growers to adopt healthier means of farming? If pesticides used by conventional growers last a long time in the environment and we encourage it, won't we be potentially affecting the safety of food supplies for years to come? Remember, genetic mutations caused by poisons can take a generation or two to rear their ugly heads. Will our grandchildren appreciate the world we created for them? However, if we demand more wholesome means of food production by voting in the grocery line by buying organic food whenever possible, won't that drive growers and food manufacturers to want to produce more organic foods? We *can* demand a healthier world by consistently sending a message through our buying habits.

On the other hand, I do realize that many readers are on a tight budget, where every penny counts. In that case, there are certain foods that I can strongly encourage you to buy organic. The Environmental Working Group (EWG) is a nonprofit organization devoted to protecting the most vulnerable segments of the human population (babies, children, and infants in the womb) from the health problems that can be attributed to toxic contaminants. They strive to replace government policies that damage the environment with conservational policies that encourage sustainable development. Their website (http://www.ewg.org/ foodnews/) lists the "Dirty Dozen Plus" foods, that should be purchased organic whenever possible, as well as the "Clean 15" foods that are known to be the lowest in pesticide.

Whether or not you choose to buy organic foods, the best way to minimize pesticide and bacteria exposure is by thoroughly washing the food. I recommend washing it in your filtered water. For foods that are scrub-able (i.e., those foods that will not be ruined by taking a hard scrubbing brush to them), I recommend you scrub them thoroughly. For foods that cannot tolerate scrubbing, such as berries, I recommend washing them at least three times in filtered water. For example, place the food in a mixing bowl, cover with water, agitate with clean hands, drain into a colander, and repeat at least two more times. After that, rinse well in the colander to get any final residue off. The old saying is "If it rains off, it drains off," and it is applicable in many areas of medicine.

For a Homework exercise, please go to http://www.ewg.org, and find the "Dirty Dozen Plus" and "Clean 15." Educate your spouse, your children, and your friends about your plan to minimize pesticide contamination. Inform them of the state of the food world with respect to exposure to genetically modified foods. Discuss what your buying habits will be in the future. Encourage your family and friends to educate others; create a ripple effect!

PART 3:
Let's Dive In!

GETTING PREPARED

Now that we have addressed the basics of your health assessment and the basics of your nutritional needs, it is time to get to the fun basics of becoming 95% (or more) vegan! You are about to begin to take full control of your nutritional health. Doesn't that feel great? It is also going to be fun to discover this world of delicious plant-based dining. Enjoy the ride!

Although it might be optimal for us all to eat only raw whole foods, the reality is that we need to put together satisfying meals for our families and ourselves in order to maintain our vegan lifestyle long-term. This is where the vegan cookbooks and your own kitchen creativity come into play. Personally, I could not imagine *never* having some of the comfort foods I love, such as macaroni and cheese, some stews, and delicious pasta dishes. The good news is that we have brilliant vegan chefs out there who have figured out how to make suitable meat-free and dairy-free substitutes of these favorites, and they have written cookbooks for the rest of us!

If you have never made anything from a written recipe before, take heart. You probably do a lot of things in your life much more complicated than following a recipe, so I know you can get the hang of this. All you need to start is a set of measuring cups and spoons and perhaps some bowls for mixing larger quantities of food. If a recipe calls for one cup of flour, spoon the flour into the one cup measurement and scrape any excess off the top so that the flour is even with the top of the cup. Do not pack the flour in; gently spoon in and level. Do the same thing with measuring spoons—scrape any excess off the top so that your measure follows the recipe exactly. If there are terms in the recipe you don't understand, there are plenty of resources, including the internet, which can show you exactly how to carry out the instruction.

It is important that you take all the time you need to feel fully prepared to adopt this new way of eating. Starting off unprepared can cause you to feel that you are failing. For example, if you don't take the time to do the Homework assignments in this section and just go off buying and eating spinach salads and grapes, what will happen when you really have a hankering for some comfort food? You won't be prepared and may go off on the binge that leaves you feeling guilty and unsuccessful. There is no rush; go at your own pace, but do go in the right direction *consistently*.

KITCHEN EQUIPMENT

Remember, an important message of this book is that you do not have to be perfect to be successful. If you cannot afford or don't have the space to buy a piece of equipment that sounds like a good idea, there are *always* old-fashioned solutions to what these machines do. Assuming you already have the basics—pots, pans, measuring cups and spoons, a hand mixer, knives for cutting produce and bread, a rolling pin, plates, cups, glasses, and silverware—you are pretty good to go as far as getting started. For many vegan recipes, you will find that having a blender and a food processor makes preparation a breeze.

Once you have your blender and food processor, you can start to consider other equipment that will make your life easier such as:

- A mincer for fresh garlic and ginger. It not only makes it easier than to mince by hand, it also releases more of the flavor of the food.

- An upright mixer. It is just so nice to be able to walk away and do other things while the mixer takes care of the mixing.

- A rice cooker. If you are like me, you have burned dozens of pots making rice and hate the sticky, gooey mess on the bottom of the pot. A rice cooker solves all of your rice problems and makes a perfect batch every time.

- A sprouting jar. Don't get nervous. I realize this likely conjures up mental images of hippies in bandanas. I must admit I was initially intimidated by the thought of sprouting. The cookbook *Vegan Artisan Cheese* (see Appendix 1) inspired me to try so that I could make the incredible recipes for more realistic cheeses. It is quite easy to do, so don't be intimidated. You can use a regular quart-sized glass jar with cheesecloth, but a sprouting jar comes with a screw-on screen top. This saves money in the long run.

- A small electric handy chopper. This is sort of a food processor to chop smaller quantities of nuts or other food that the larger food processor can't reach.

- A bread machine with a timer feature. You can just make bread and pizza dough much faster with a machine. Also, if you buy one with a timer, you can put all of the ingredients in the machine and time it to be done just when you wake up in the morning or get home from work in the evening.

- A slow cooker (Crock-Pot®). Especially for soups and stews in which you are using dried, soaked peas or beans, it makes for simple preparation and easy cleanup.

- A masticating juicer. We will discuss this more in depth below.

- A meat slicer. If you make seitan that is to be sliced thin to put on sandwiches, a meat slicer will make it much easier to do. If you don't care about having thinly sliced deli meat, you do not need a meat slicer.

Remember, the equipment is just a luxury for faster preparation and convenience. Don't let not having the equipment stop you from striving to be 95% vegan.

THE BASICS OF VEGAN COOKING

Most of us grew up with the following four food groups: meat and dairy, fruits, vegetables, and grains. Your new four food groups as a vegan are nuts and legumes, grains, fruits and vegetables.

You will simply be amazed at how simple and delicious vegan fare can be. You will also likely find that many of the foods you were already enjoying are already vegan or can become vegan with just a minor adjustment or two. Celine Steen and Joni Marie Newman's book *The Complete Guide to Vegan Food Substitutions* is an invaluable resource to help you convert non-vegan recipes into equally wonderful vegan fare. Also, be sure to peruse Appendix 1 for our other favorite cookbooks.

Another inexpensive option to start would be to visit your local library and borrow some vegan cookbooks. This way, you can try out some recipes from these books, and decide which ones you may want to buy. Vegan cooking can be as simple or as complicated as you want it to be. I personally found a lot of joy discovering, and in some cases, rediscovering various spices and herbs, as well as cooking methods, while reducing the fat in our meals.

In vegan recipes, you will discover there are many ingredients that you never would have thought would find their way into your shopping cart. Some you may not be familiar with (such as nutritional yeast flakes, vital wheat gluten, and tempeh) and others you didn't think were for cooking (maple syrup, for example). Yet you will find these items become new staples in your pantry.

At first glance at some of the recipes in vegan cookbooks, I remember thinking, *oh great, I have to get the food processor out. It's going to be a big job.* The recipes looked intimidating and messy, even to me as a dietitian. However, I quickly found that with a few pulses with a blender or food processor, I had a meal that was far more delicious than anything I had ever eaten as an omnivore. As I became more familiar with vegan cooking, I also got faster at it. My advice is to not allow yourself to be intimidated, know that you are simply on a learning curve, and things will get easier the more you do them.

I also learned to appreciate the value of tofu—yes, I said it. Tofu: that thing we all say we hate though few of us even know what to do with it. I will admit that it took about a year before I really learned to enjoy it. Many vegan recipes call for tofu (and many do not). Oftentimes, the purpose of the tofu is similar to that of eggs, cheese, or cream; you don't necessarily taste these ingredients in the recipe, but they are there for a purpose, such as eggs being used an emulsifier or binding agent. They are not there for their own flavor. Once I started cooking with tofu, I became much less wary of it, to the point in where I now enjoy many dishes in which tofu is the star of the show. Try to keep an open mind when it comes to tofu. I highly recommend you buy or borrow from your local library one or two cookbooks that will have excellent recipes to initiate you to cooking with it.

Seitan (pronounced *say-tan*) is what is known as vegan meat. It is usually made with vital wheat gluten, nutritional yeast flakes, and seasonings, such as soy sauce, a vegan broth, or a product called Bragg Liquid Aminos®. These ingredients will become permanent fixtures in your pantry. In my opinion, seitan is usually more flavorful than its meat counterparts and has an easier texture to chew. What I have found is that I can make seitan in quantities and freeze it. Thus, I only have to make it once or twice a month. I usually make chicken, beef, and turkey seitan. I also sometimes make more adventurous seitan such as Cajun-spiced. What is really nice about it is that, relative to meat, seitan is quite inexpensive. One thing I would like to make you aware of is the fact that many seitan recipes call for using plain water. The Better than Bouillon® product line has "No Beef" and "No Chicken" mixtures which are delicious and really do taste like the meat variety. Using these instead of plain water makes for a more flavorful seitan recipe, in my opinion.

Tempeh is another meat substitute, but you will buy it, not make it at home. It is a complicated thing to make, as it requires fermentation, so it is easier to just buy it when a recipe you want to try calls for it.

You will find yourself looking for sales on nuts, especially cashews. They are used very frequently in all types of recipes. One of my favorite recipes is a carrot cake with a cream cheese frosting, made with cashew butter. It is so amazing what vegan chefs have come up with to make such yummy meat and dairy-alternative dishes. Thank goodness for all of the cookbooks they have published!

For those days when you need quick hot meals for dinner, you can always buy ready-made vegan burgers, pizza, and TV dinners. I also like to make my own pizza using vegan pizza dough (available commercially but can also be made easily in a bread maker), some type of vegan cheese, fresh or frozen vegetables, sun-dried tomatoes, and homemade sauce. I freeze them so that I have quick meals on-hand, making the pizza myself in advance also saves money.

There are many vegan substitutes commercially available now for cheese, yogurt, hotdogs, sausages, etc. Some of them are very good, and many are not. Some of them are very high in sodium. And most of them are far more expensive than if I make them myself at home. I have not really found a good, hard cheese substitute in which I like both the product and the nutritional information (some are quite high in fat). I do sometimes like to buy the sausage substitutes to put on my pizza or in a pasta sauce. I encourage you to read the label before you buy anything to ensure it is not too high in sodium for you, and of course, watch the fat. More and more soy yogurt products are entering the market at a blistering pace. Some are better than others; you will have to decide for yourself on these products since individual tastes vary so much.

Another avenue for finding wonderful vegan fare is to scope out the Asian grocery stores and markets, if they are available in your area. They have become my replacement for fast-food chains. Many creative, pre-made dishes and desserts are available at astonishing prices.

As you gain confidence, you will discover many, many wonderful ways to prepare delicious and nutritious meals. Don't forget to see Appendix 1 for suggested resources, and have fun!

THE POWER OF JUICING

Juicing at home using a masticating juicer is a great way to get concentrated nutrition quickly. The concentrated juice contains huge quantities of antioxidants and other valuable nutrients. It is a great way to get a low-calorie, nutritious meal without cooking! Because it is made with raw, whole fruits and vegetables, it is much more nutritious than most commercially prepared juices. Be aware that fresh juices should either be consumed on the day you have juiced them, or you can add a very small quantity of ascorbic acid crystals or lemon juice and refrigerate for a few days.

Myth: It doesn't matter whether you juice at home or buy juice in the store.

Fact: Most store-bought juice has either been made from concentrate, has added sugars, or has other added chemicals. All of these make the juice less healthy than a homemade glass of juice—just be sure to clean your fruits and vegetables before juicing them!

One of my favorite resources is *The Big Book of Juices* by Natalie Savona, published by Duncan Baird Publishers. It has a wide range of recipes for delicious juice concoctions as well as smoothies.

Another wonderful thing I have found about juicing is that it is a great way to use fresh fruits and vegetables that I find I will not have the time to eat or cook but don't want to waste. I have invented many interesting juices this way. Sometimes a splash of Tabasco® or other flavoring is all that is needed to turn an otherwise bland juice into something wonderful.

I mentioned earlier that I recommend a masticating juicer. Masticating juicers basically chew fruits and vegetables to squeeze out the juice retaining more of the nutrients and flavor. They are more versatile than centrifugal juicers (spinning juicers) in that they can juice leafy greens, such as kale, much better. They can also be used to make nut butters. They are uncomplicated and easy to clean. While they tend to be more expensive than the centrifugal juicers, you can find very good prices at online retailers such as Amazon.

When it comes to juicing, there are really no rules. Be creative, enjoy the tremendous nutrition, and have fun!

READING LABELS
FOR VEGANISM

• •

Reading labels to ensure a product is 100 percent vegan is an important step to ensure you stay 95% vegan. If you are allowing yourself to eat one meat- and/or dairy-containing meal per week, then it is important that you ensure the rest of your week is 100 percent vegan to achieve 95% for that week overall.

You may find that some of the things you have really enjoyed were already vegan. I had that experience. Confession: my guilty food pleasures include Oreos® and Cap'n Crunch® cereal. And guess what? I discovered that neither one of them contain any animal products! I only buy them very rarely because neither are what I'd call valuable food, but it's nice to know that when I need to give in to the craving, the vegan part of my diet is still taken care of.

On many labels, you will see that while the product itself is vegan, there is a notice that the product was manufactured in a plant that also processes milk and other animal products. If you have severe allergies to any of the products processed in the plant, you certainly want to avoid that product. Some vegans will not buy these products based on their principles of not wanting to support any businesses that engage in working with animal products. If either of these two scenarios applies to you, then it is a quick decision to steer clear of that product.

Another product that hardcore vegans will not eat is honey because honeybees, which are animals, make it for us. Since I engage in veganism mostly for health reasons, I do not worry about eating honey as it does not contain any of the proteins or fats found in animal products. Of course, the decision is a personal one you will have to make for yourself.

Many commercial products now have it clearly marked on the packaging if the product is vegan.

A quick way to tell if a product is made without dairy is to look for the word *pareve* or *parve* on the container. This is a label used by Jewish people to ensure they will not accidentally eat meat with dairy, which is prohibited by Jewish law. Pareve products will usually have this symbol:

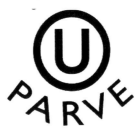

Beyond obvious markings of a product being vegan, you will need to read the ingredients label to determine for yourself if the product is vegan. The good thing is that this is relatively simple as most non-vegan ingredients are readily identifiable. Eggs, milk, milk solids, milk fat, lard, and cream are all obvious animal products. Some less obvious animal-containing products are whey, casein, and gelatin. Vegan gelatin exists, but since companies tend to list "gelatin" as an ingredient without further explanation, you can assume that it is animal-based. Then there is the occasionally confusing ingredient such as cream of tartar. Does the word *cream* mean it is of animal origin? No. Cream of tartar is a chemical called potassium hydrogen tartrate and does not come from an animal source. Another one is malt since many people think of malted milk when they hear the word. Malt is actually a grain product. Malted milk products are not vegan. However, you can buy barley malt if you want to enjoy making an old-fashioned malted milk drink vegan (Of course, you will need to mix it with a nondairy milk product.). Cocoa butter (also called "cacao butter") is also not of animal origin but from cocoa beans, however you should only use food grade cocoa butter for cooking.

You will likely begin to notice ingredients in which you never thought about their origin, animal-based or not. Depending on how hardcore vegan you want to be, some ingredients used as thickeners can be technically considered animal product sources because they are made by fermenting sugars by bacteria (which some people think of as an animal because it is a living organism). Xanthan gum is one example of this, although some vegan cookbooks do call for it. I personally do not worry about this since the product does not add any animal protein or fat. You choose for yourself; there is no wrong answer since xanthan gum doesn't add any meat or dairy nutritive value. If you do want to stick with plant-based thickeners, Irish Moss (from which carrageenan is made), guar gum, agar, cornstarch, pectin, and flours all fall into that category.

Label reading for veganism is quite simple, once you know these basics. However, if you are not familiar with a specific ingredient, you may want to read up on it before buying it. A quick Google search will usually tell you exactly what you need to know.

Your First Steps

Now that you have read the basics of becoming prepared, it is time for you to put some first steps into action.

Homework

1. Go to Appendix 1 to review the suggest resources. Many cookbooks are listed. Choose just one, the one that interests you the most. You can either purchase the book at the retailer of your choice or see if you can borrow it from your local library. If none of the listed books are available at your library and you are not ready to purchase one, find a vegan cookbook that is available at the library and borrow that one instead.

2. Choose two recipes that interest you from the vegan cookbook. I encourage you to make one of your choices a main meal you have never had before, but that sounds tasty to you. The other one can be whatever else you think is interesting.

3. Make a grocery list of the items you will need to buy in order to make the two recipes.

4. If the grocery list contains items that you cannot find in your local grocery store, consider visiting a Whole Foods®, Fresh Market®, Trader Joe's®, or a farmers market. You can also Google the items by typing "buy" and the item in question, example "buy Vital Wheat Gluten." This will list online retailers from which you can purchase the item. Oftentimes, you will find this to be the less expensive option anyway. You don't have to spend the gas money to find the items at various stores; the items are often less expensive in non-brick-and-mortar stores, and you can often get free shipping too.

5. Once you have all of the ingredients, commit time to make the recipes.

6. Make serving up this new lifestyle fun for yourself and your family. Perhaps you can serve it on your best dinnerware, garnish the plates however you wish, use cocktail glasses for water or other beverage, or make it into a fun picnic. Even if it is winter in New Hampshire, you can lay down a tablecloth in your living room and have a wonderful time!

95% VEGAN ON A BUDGET

I can't tell you how many patients have told me they cannot afford to go vegan because of the expense of fruit and vegetables. I can certainly relate to a concern about large grocery bills. However, I can also relate to those huge medical expenses and the human toll that accompanies the ravages of diabetes, heart disease, and cancer and can truly tell you that the investment to prevent these diseases is worth it. If you have a perception that your grocery bill will be higher than the grocery bills you have now, I believe you will be pleasantly surprised by the facts.

Your need for protein will be met by foods high in lysine: beans and legumes. Whether they are used in a unique recipe or eaten plain, they are certainly less expensive than meat counterparts. The main increase in cost for veganism does lie in the expense for fruit and vegetables. You likely didn't get all of the servings of fruits and vegetables for optimal health before because 90 percent of the U.S. population doesn't. You just weren't hungry for them because you were so satiated by less healthy options, including fast foods. So the expense for more fruits and vegetables will offset the savings from buying less expensive protein sources. However, if we consider that we also eat far too many calories for good health, it becomes clear that we don't need to buy huge quantities of fruits and vegetables to meet our healthy caloric needs. Three to five servings of fruit and four to six servings of non-starchy vegetables (starchy vegetables include corn, potatoes, and peas) daily are sufficient for the majority of adults. What you have eaten in the past for fruit and vegetables is fine; you will just be eating more of them now.

LET'S COMPARE, SHALL WE?

. . . .

One of the biggest myths about the vegan diet (as well as eating healthy in general) is that it is too expensive to maintain. Many believe that they simply cannot afford to follow a vegan diet. Another general concern is that a vegan diet does not provide all of the nutrients a person needs, especially protein. In this chapter, we're going to bust these myths! Not only can a vegan diet be less expensive than a comparable omnivore diet, but it can also be much healthier while providing the nutrients we need.

In this chapter, I will show you comparable seven-day meal plans for both a vegan and a non-vegan diet. The items each day at each meal are comparable between the two diets. For example, one day the breakfast for both is a bagel with cream cheese; however, the vegan breakfast calls for vegan cream cheese substitutes. I did this to demonstrate how a vegan diet does not require you to radically alter your daily choices. I also wanted to be fair in showing the costs and nutritional comparisons between the vegan and omnivore diet to give you as clear a picture as possible. But before you see the chart of the seven-day meal plans, let's first go over some of the symbols and measurements we used.

Symbol	Meaning
*	Indicates an original recipe, located in Appendix 5
†	Indicates a recipe from an outside source, cited in the chapter references
V.	Vegan

For the sake of space, I do not list every item in the vegan portion of the spreadsheet as vegan. I opt instead to use "V". to designate a vegan food. However, everything in the "Vegan" portion of the spreadsheet is vegan, regardless of whether its name makes it sound like a non-vegan food. For example, the sour cream and mayo in the Vegan Day 1 are vegan substitutes. Some of the vegan recipes such as the V. Biscuit and V. Ghiradelli® Brownie are adapted from non-vegan recipes. In the Ghiradelli® Brownie, I substituted one tablespoon ground flaxseed and three tablespoons of water for the egg in the recipe printed on the side of the brownie mix box. In the V. Biscuit, I used vegetable shortening and either soymilk or water rather than butter and dairy milk.

Each day both the vegan and non-vegan meal plans contain a breakfast, lunch, dinner, and dessert. The calculations of their nutrition and costs are based upon the cost and nutrition of the entire recipe divided by however much is in a portion size. For example, the chick'n seitan recipe creates about a pound of seitan, so divide that by 16 to get the nutrition and cost per ounce and then multiply those numbers by 3 because the serving in the table is three ounces. Simple enough, right?

You will see that some vegan items in the chart are more expensive than their animal-based counterparts. Soymilk will be more expensive than dairy milk per cup, for example. In fact, some entire vegan diet days are more expensive than their non-vegan counterparts. But you will also see that some vegan items, especially homemade meat substitutes are much less expensive than meats. Just hold on until the end of the chapter before you come to any conclusions about the cost and nutrition of the vegan diet. You will see that overall the vegan diet is less expensive, contains less fat, has adequate protein, and is just as delicious as the non-vegan diet. Without any further ado, I give you the seven-day meal plan spreadsheet.

		DAY 1	$ per serving	Cals	Fat	Pro	Carb	Fiber
Non-Vegan Meal Plan	Breakfast	Cheerios®, 1cup	$0.22	100	2	3	20	3
		2% milk, 1 cup	$0.22	122	5	8	12	0
	Lunch	2 slices wheat bread	$0.25	140	3	8	26	4
		2 oz deli roast beef	$1.44	90	3	15	0	0
		2 oz deli swiss cheese	$1.00	220	18	14	1	0
		1 tbsp mayonnaise	$0.08	90	10	0	0	0
		potato chips, 1 oz	$0.41	150	10	2	15	1
	Dinner	Burrito: 4oz ground beef w/ onion and spices	$0.62	558	40	24	0	0
		sour cream, 2 tbp	$0.18	58	5	1	2	0
		shredded cheese, 2 oz	$0.90	226	18	7	0	0
		tortilla, lettuce, tomato	$0.52	160	4	4	28	1
	Dessert	fruit popsicle	$0.78	80	0	0	19	1
	Total		$6.62	1994	118	86	123	10
Vegan Meal Plan	Breakfast	Cheerios®, 1cup	$0.22	100	2	3	20	3
		vanilla soy milk, 1 cup	$0.38	100	3.5	6	11	1
	Lunch	2 slices wheat bread	$0.25	140	3	8	26	4
		Pastrami Seitan†, 2 oz	$0.40	130	4	18	8	2
		V. havarti spread, 1/4 c.	$0.40	138	6	8	17	4
		V. mayo	0.1	90	9	0	0	0
		potato chips, 1 oz	0.41	150	10	2	15	1
	Dinner	Mexicali TVP*, 1 serving	$0.68	235	8	25	17	10
		V. sour cream, 2 tbsp	$0.22	60	5.5	2	3	0
		Melty White Cheez†, 1/4 cup	$0.51	85	3	5	11	1
		tortilla, lettuce, tomato	$0.52	160	4	4	28	1
	Dessert	fruit popsicle	$0.78	80	0	0	19	1
	Total		$4.87	1468	58	81	175	28

		DAY 2	$ per serving	Cals	Fat	Pro	Carb	Fiber
Non-Vegan Meal Plan	Breakfast	cinnamon raisin bagel	$0.33	290	2	10	57	4
		cream cheese, 2 tbsp	$0.24	100	9	2	1	0
	Lunch	2 tbsp vinaigrette	$0.22	90	9	0	3	0
		large veggie salad	$1.50	164	1	10	35	15
		1 egg	$0.15	71	5	6	0	0
		turkey, 2 oz	$1.25	60	0	10	2	0
		deli cheddar, 1 oz	$0.60	113	9	7	0	0
	Dinner	spaghetti, 1 c, cooked	$0.15	220	1	8	43	3
		meatballs, 4 oz	$0.79	300	22	16	8	0
		tomato sauce, 1/2 c	$0.58	70	2	2	12	3
		mozzarella, 2 oz	$0.70	168	12	12	2	0
	Dessert	3 small spritz cookies	$0.16	204	12	2	23	3
	Total		**$6.67**	**1850**	**84**	**85**	**186**	**28**
Vegan Meal Plan	Breakfast	cinnamon raisin bagel	$0.33	290	2	10	57	4
		V. cream cheese, 2 tbsp	$0.41	90	9	1	1	0
	Lunch	skillet biscuit*, 1 serving	$0.55	163	3	9	24	3
		large veggie salad	$1.50	164	1	10	35	15
		2 tbsp vinaigrette	$0.22	90	9	0	3	0
	Dinner	spaghetti, 1 c, cooked	$0.15	220	1	8	43	3
		Italian TVP*, 1 serving	$0.68	235	8	25	17	10
		tomato sauce, 1/2 c	$0.56	70	2	2	12	3
		Fresh Mozzarella†, 1/4 c	$0.94	108	8	3	6	1
	Dessert	3 Vegan Spritz Cookies*	$0.16	201	12	2	23	3
	Total		**$5.50**	**1631**	**55**	**70**	**221**	**42**

		DAY 3	$ per serving	Cals	Fat	Pro	Carb	Fiber
Non-Vegan Meal Plan	Breakfast	oatmeal, cooked, 1 cup	$0.14	166	4	6	32	4
		brown sugar, 1 tbsp	$0.09	51	0	0	12	0
		coffee, half & half 1/4c	0.16	80	6	2	2	0
	Lunch	Subway® 6-inch Cold Cut Combo sandwich	$3.75	370	13	18	46	5
		potato chips, 1 oz	0.41	150	10	2	15	1
	Dinner	Chicken breast, 3 oz cooked	$0.65	142	3	27	0	0
		green peas, 1 c	$0.45	134	0	9	25	9
		cooked rice, 1 c	$0.24	205	0	4	45	1
		mixed vegetables, 1 c	$0.30	110	0	6	24	8
	Dessert	Blackberry cobbler (1/8)	$1.51	377	10	6.5	69	8
	Total		**$7.70**	**1785**	**46**	**80.5**	**270**	**36**
Vegan Meal Plan	Breakfast	oatmeal, cooked, 1 cup	$0.14	166	4	6	32	4
		brown sugar, 1 tbsp	$0.09	51	0	0	12	0
		coffee, 1 c soy milk	0.38	100	3.5	6	11	1
	Lunch	Subway® 6-inch Veggie Delight sandwich	$3.75	230	2.5	8	44	5
		potato chips, 1 oz	0.41	150	10	2	15	1
	Dinner	Chick'n Seitan* 3oz	$0.73	180	5.5	48	15	2
		green peas, 1 c	$0.45	134	0	9	25	9
		cooked rice, 1 c	$0.24	205	0	4	45	1
		mixed vegetables, 1 c	$0.30	110	0	6	24	8
	Dessert	Blackberry Grunt† (1/8)	$1.53	372	10	6	69	8
	Total		**$8.02**	**1698**	**35.5**	**95**	**292**	**39**

		DAY 4	$ per serving	Cals	Fat	Pro	Carb	Fiber
Non-Vegan Meal Plan	Breakfast	toast, 2 slices	$0.25	140	3	8	26	4
		1 tbsp butter	$0.09	101	11.5	0	0	0
	Lunch	Moe's chicken burrito (with black beans, guaca-mole, sour cream, and vegetables)	$7.19	880	47.5	35	50	3
	Dinner	hamburger bun	$0.31	180	2.5	7	36	2
		hamburger, 4 oz cooked	$0.47	558	40	24	0	0
		American cheese, slice	$0.19	60	5	3	1	0
		ketchup, 2 tbsp	$0.12	27	0	0	7	0
		steamed broccoli, 1 c	$0.30	54	0	2	6	3
	Dessert	ice cream sandwich	$0.33	160	5	2	25	0
	Total		**$9.25**	**2160**	**115**	**81**	**151**	**12**
Vegan Meal Plan	Breakfast	toast, 2 slices	$0.25	140	3	8	26	4
		1 tbsp V. butter	$0.13	100	11	0	0	0
	Lunch	Moe's bean bur-rito (with black beans, guaca-mole, sour cream, and vegetables)	$5.99	720	31	22	87	12
	Dinner	hamburger bun	$0.31	180	2.5	7	36	2
		2 store-bought veggie burgers	$1.84	240	3	36	18	12
		Soft Gruyere†, 1 oz	$0.50	142	12	4	6	1
		ketchup, 2 tbsp	$0.12	27	0	0	7	0
		steamed broccoli, 1 c	$0.30	54	0	2	6	3
	Dessert	V. ice cream sandwich	$0.95	130	6	2	17	0
	Total		**$10.39**	**1733**	**68.5**	**81**	**203**	**34**

		DAY 5	$ per serving	Cals	Fat	Pro	Carb	Fiber
Non-Vegan Meal Plan	Breakfast	yogurt, 6 fl. oz.	$0.75	170	1.5	5	33	0
		granola, 1/4 c	$0.29	85	1	2.5	17	1.5
		blueberries, 1/2 c	0.75	42	0	0.5	10.5	2
	Lunch	baked potato, 6 oz	$0.33	161	0	4	37	4
		sour cream, 4 tbsp	0.35	116	10	2	4	0
		cheddar, 2 oz	0.9	226	18	14	0	0
		broccoli, 1/2 c	0.15	27	0	1	3	1.5
	Dinner	beef and veggie stew	$2.48	256	8	29	18	4.5
		Pillsbury® biscuit	0.19	170	6	3	25	1
	Dessert	Ghiradelli® brownie	$0.21	185	8	1	26	1
	Total		**$6.40**	**1438**	**52.5**	**62**	**173.5**	**15.5**
Vegan Meal Plan	Breakfast	V. yogurt, 6 fl. oz.	$0.87	150	3	5	25	1
		granola, 1/4 c	$0.29	85	1	2.5	17	1.5
		blueberries, 1/2 c	0.75	42	0	0.5	10.5	2
	Lunch	baked potato, 6 oz	$0.33	161	0	4	37	4
		V. sour cream, 4 tbsp	0.45	126	11	4	6	1
		Sharp Cheddar†, 2 oz	1.38	234	16	10	12	1
		broccoli, 1/2 c	0.19	27	0	1	3	1.5
	Dinner	bean and veggie stew*	$1.34	155	0.5	7	32	12
		V. biscuit	0.14	220	12	3	23	1
	Dessert	V. Ghiradelli® brownie	0.21	182	8	1	26	1
	Total		**$5.95**	**1382**	**51.5**	**38**	**191.5**	**26**

		DAY 6	$ per serving	Cals	Fat	Pro	Carb	Fiber
Non-Vegan Meal Plan	Breakfast	Bisquick® pancakes, 1 serving	$0.23	200	4	7	35	1
		maple syrup, 2 tbsp	$0.11	104	0	0	26	0
	Lunch	strawberry, banana, & yogurt smoothie	$1.72	348	1	5	8	2
	Dinner	Pizza Hut® large Veggie Lover's pizza, 2 slices	$3.41	660	30	26	76	4
	Dessert	mint chocolate chip ice cream, 1/2 c	$0.99	170	10	3	18	0
	Total		$6.46	1482	45	41	163	7
Vegan Meal Plan	Breakfast	Easy Vegan Pancakes*, 1 serving	$0.26	190	4	5	34	1.5
		maple syrup, 2 tbsp	$0.11	104	0	0	26	0
	Lunch	strawberry, banana, & V. yogurt smoothie	$1.79	336	2	5	77	9
	Dinner	Easy Vegan Pizza*, (1/4)	$2.13	620	24	15	84	7
	Dessert	Soy Dream® mint chocolate chip ice cream, 1/2 c	1.17	150	8	1	20	1
	Total		$5.46	1400	38	26	241	18.5

		DAY 7	$ per serving	Cals	Fat	Pro	Carb	Fiber
Non-Vegan **Meal Plan**	Breakfast	bacon, 1 oz cooked	$0.75	151	12	10	0	0
		3 eggs	$0.45	213	15	18	0	0
		2 oz shredded cheese	$0.90	226	18	14	0	0
		flaxseed oil, 1 tbsp	$0.52	119	14	0	0	0
	Lunch	Macaroni and cheese casserole, 1 cup	$0.62	460	28	18	36	2
	Dinner	pot roast, 5 oz	$2.14	240	13	21	9	3
		steamed carrots, 1 c	$0.30	54	0	2	12	4
		canned peas, 1c	$0.45	134	0	9	25	9
	Dessert	German chocolate cake (1/12 slice)	$0.41	441	24	5	53	1
	Total		**$6.54**	**2038**	**124**	**97**	**135**	**19**
Vegan **Meal Plan**	Breakfast	Tempeh Bacon†, 1 oz	$0.56	82	4	6.5	5	3
		Tofu Omelette* (contains vegan cheddar)	$3.19	570	31	29	48	8
	Lunch	Macaroni and Cheez†, 1 cup	$0.76	368	9	17	55	6
	Dinner	Pot Roast†, 1 serving	$1.08	214	8	29	13	2
		steamed carrots, 1 c	$0.30	54	0	2	12	4
		canned peas, 1c	$0.45	134	0	9	25	9
	Dessert	V. German chocolate cake (1/12 slice)	$0.42	425	23	3	54	1
	Total		**$6.76**	**1847**	**75**	**95.5**	**212**	**33**

Now let's jump straight to the punch line and compare the week's totals. The totals are rounded to the nearest whole numbers, except for the costs.

Categories	Vegan Week	Non-Vegan Week
Total Cost	$46.95	$49.64
Average Daily Cost	$6.70	$7.09
Total Calories For The Week	11001	12747
Average Calories Per Day	1572 (round to 1600)	1821 (round to 1800)
Body Weight Supported By The Above Daily Calories	105 pounds	121 pounds
Total Fat For The Week	366 grams	584 grams
Average Fat Per Day	52 grams	84 grams
Percent Of Daily Calories From Fat	30%	41%
Total Protein	480 grams	533 grams
Average Protein Per Day	69 grams	76 grams
Total Lysine For The Week	20,337 milligrams	---
Average Lysine Per Day	**2905 milligrams**	---

You may have questions about the information contained in the above table. Even though each weekly meal plan consumes roughly the same items and volume, the vegan substitutions contain inherently fewer calories. Based on the caloric intake for both plans, the vegan plan at rounded to 1,600 calories per day would support a forty- to forty-five-year-old woman between 110 and 120 pounds. The non-vegan plan rounded to 1,800 calories a day would support that forty- to forty-five-year-old woman at a weight 140–150 pounds. This is a dramatic difference, and if that forty- to forty-five-year-old woman who weighed 140–150 pounds on a non-vegan diet desired to lose weight and eat a healthier diet, switching to the vegan meal plan would do it!

But suppose that woman had a healthy BMI weighing 140–150 pounds; she might not want to lose weight. In that case, just switching to the vegan meal plan outlined here may not provide enough calories for her to maintain her current weight.

Essentially, if you don't want to lose weight while converting to a vegan diet, you would also need to increase portion sizes to make up the difference in calories because the vegan items are inherently lower in calories. Or instead of increasing portion sizes, you could increase your intake of fruits and vegetables, which would likely be an even healthier option.

"Wouldn't that cost more?" you might ask. The truth is that yes, per calorie, the vegan diet is marginally more expensive. I'm going to do some math here, but if you want to skip down to the punch line, you can do that too.

To begin with, on the non-vegan meal plan, we already know that it costs $7.09 a day to have roughly 1,800 non-vegan calories. The vegan meal plan costs $6.70 a day for 1,600 calories. But if a person wanted to follow a similar vegan meal plan that amounted to 1,800 calories, it would cost $7.54 a day. The difference then is $0.45 a day to switch from 1,800 non-vegan calories to 1,800 vegan calories a day. Here's how we get to that figure:

$6.70 ÷ 1600 calories = $0.00419 per calorie

$0.00419 x 1,800 calories = $7.54 for 1,800 calories each day on a vegan diet.

$7.54 (for 1,800 vegan calories per day) – $7.09 (for 1,800 non vegan calories per day) = $0.45 per day difference between 1,800 non-vegan and vegan calories.

So whether a vegan diet is more or less expensive than a non-vegan diet comes down to how you look at it. If you want to lose weight but consume roughly the same food items (as I suspect many people do), then vegan comes out to be less expensive; you eat the same items at a lower cost. If you are already at a healthy weight while being an omnivore and want to go vegan while maintaining the same number of calories per day, then vegan is more expensive by about $0.45 a day based on the meal plan provided. Even so, there are two things you should consider along with this information: (1) You can cut costs on the vegan diet in ways that I did not account for in this meal plan such as following sales, coupon-clipping, or shopping at discount grocery stores, and (2) you should compare any extra cost of the vegan diet to the costs associated with the health issues associated with obesity and the consumption of animal products.

In the vegan week meal plan, I included some pre-prepared food items as well as restaurant items in an attempt to mimic the average American's diet and habits. For example, some days running to the sandwich shop for lunch is easier if you were running late for work and couldn't pack a meal. However, that restaurant option is more expensive; if you instead were to pack the vegan pastrami-style seitan sandwich, it would save a couple of dollars. Similarly, you could make your own vegan hamburger patties from TVP, and that would be less expensive than the prepared frozen veggie burgers.

You can also order many vegan substitute items in bulk at discounted rates online. Amazon.com and vitacost.com carry many vegan items, such as TVP (texturized vegetable protein), and will ship cases of the items at a rate much lower than you might find in a specialty grocery store. Many vegan items do not spoil as quickly as non-vegan items; you can keep TVP in your pantry or freezer for long periods, long after comparable ground beef would have spoiled. The point is that if you are a savvy shopper, you can follow a vegan diet at a discount while becoming nutritionally healthier and not sacrificing any quality!

Eating a healthy vegan diet *might* add some expense to your grocery bills. However, the money you may save with reduced medication or supplement needs, as well as by warding off chronic illnesses, make the vegan diet an economically viable plan. For a small-scale example, the vegan diet can help reduce levels of LDL, so if you're taking a statin, you might find you can lower the dosage to meet your target or you may no longer need it. A more significant example is a heart attack; the vegan diet has been proven to help prevent and reverse heart disease and can help you avoid other serious health problems. Consider that a hospital's costs on average to treat a heart attack was over $50,000 in 2007[1], and whatever a patient's insurance does not cover, the patient typically must pay. That does not include the cost of ongoing treatments; rehabilitation, doctor visits, medications, or lost productivity in the workplace. It also doesn't count the intangible costs of pain and suffering from the heart attack and subsequent treatment or time lost doing the things you enjoy. The old saying that "An ounce of prevention is worth a pound of cure," is evident when the vegan diet is the prevention for a heart attack or other serious illness.

Separating from the question of cost, the vegan diet is healthier than its non-vegan counterpart. By switching to vegan options, a person would reduce their intake of fat from 84 grams to 52 grams per day. This reduces the percentage of that person's calories from fat from 41 percent to 30 percent, which is an astounding amount! A maximum of 25–35 percent of a person's calories should come from fat according to the American Heart Association[2]; less fat is better. The non-vegan meal plan exceeds the recommended fat intake, while the vegan diet is squarely in safe territory.

What about protein? The vegan meal plan provides only slightly less protein than the non-vegan meal plan, but it still exceeds an average person's protein needs. And you need not worry about the quality of the protein provided by the vegan diet. The main essential amino acid of concern for vegans is lysine, which in a vegan diet is present primarily in legumes. A person's lysine needs are determined by their weight; the requirement for most people is around 30 mg per day of lysine a day per kilogram of body weight. For example, a person who is 105 pounds (48 kg) needs about 1,432 mg of lysine a day. The vegan meal plan presented in this chapter contained an average of 2,905 mg of lysine per day, well above that person's needs! The other essential amino acids are also easily covered in this week's meal plan.

In conclusion, when you trade a non-vegan diet for a vegan diet, you can lose weight, lower fat intake, maintain adequate protein, and enjoy the same types of foods you enjoyed before. While a calorically equivalent vegan diet costs roughly $0.45 more a day than a non-vegan diet, most of us need to lose weight anyway, and reducing calories while eating your favorite dishes is practically magic! Knowing what you now know about the health benefits of a vegan diet, even if it costs a few cents more a day, isn't it worth it to avoid the health consequences of the standard Western diet? I think so.

VEGAN FRUGAL FUN
BY THE SEASON

• •

Now that we have established that it is possible to follow a vegan diet without ruining the food budget, let's talk about how to make it fun! Holidays and traditional foods by the season are well ingrained in our culture for very good reason: they bring us together with those we love and create cherished memories. Let's go through the entire year and highlight just how we can make it yummy *and* vegan. Of course, you can certainly save your animal-product days for holidays, but we also encourage you to try some of the ideas and original recipes (see Appendix 5) so that you can begin to create the ripple effect for future generations. We tend to love the food with which we associate happy memories and comfort. For example, those who grew up in the north typically stuff their Thanksgiving turkey with various types of stuffing, while those who grew up in the south do not; they make cornbread dressing in an oven plate. Neither of them really grabs onto the others' tradition; they want what mama used to make! The same goes for pasta dishes. "I love my mother's lasagna, no one makes it better than her." So now *you* can affect the foods that your children and grandchildren will remember and cherish, simply by serving it to them in your loving environment. From season-to-season, you can create vegan frugal fun! Here we will highlight the major holidays celebrated in the United States. Of course, you can enjoy any of the holiday food at any time; you are not boxed in to enjoy it only on one day! The most expensive recipe is the Tres Leches cake, at 76 cents per serving. The least expensive is the Challah Bread at 25 cents per serving. As you go through each season, you will note that we haven't included some holidays you may have expected. This is because the traditional foods for those holidays are usually repeats from other holidays we did discuss. In our family, springtime is when we feel as if we are coming out of hibernation to enjoy all that nature has to offer, so we will start there. This season goes from March 21 to June 20.

Spring [March 21-June 20]

See Appendix 5 for our Ambrosia recipe and Vegan Marshmallows. The flavor brings you right out of the winter doldrums!

Spring's Seasonal Fruits and Vegetables

apples
artichokes
asparagus
avocados
broccoli
Brussels sprouts
cabbage
cauliflower
celery
chard
cherries
collards
dates
fava beans

(Spring's Seasonal Fruits and Vegetables, Cont'd)
fennel
grapefruit
jicama
kale
kumquats
leeks
lemons
lettuce
limes
Mandarin oranges
mushrooms
oranges
parsnips
pomelos
potatoes
radishes
scallions
shallots
strawberries
tangerines
turnips

St. Patrick's Day

Saint Patrick's Day commemorates the death of Saint Patrick, believed to have been on March 17, 461. Saint Patrick is credited with bringing Christianity to Ireland and explaining the Holy Trinity using the three leaves on a shamrock. In the United States, the holiday is now largely a celebration of Irish heritage and includes parades, consuming green-colored food and beer, and other festivities. There are a number of dishes traditionally eaten on St. Patrick's Day in the United States, including corned beef, cabbage, and Irish soda bread. These dishes are not necessarily authentic to Ireland, but they're what we typically eat in the United States to celebrate the holiday. For more information, visit http://www.history.com/topics/st-patricks-day. See Appendix 5 for original Corned Beef and Irish Soda Bread recipes.

Earth Day

The first governmentally sanctioned Earth Day was held April 22, 1970. Nationwide demonstrations against the degradation of the environment were held. The protests led to the creation of the EPA and passage of the Clean Air, Clean Water, and Endangered Species Acts. Today, Earth Day is celebrated by performing environmentally aware actions such as planting a tree, pledging an act of green, or having a picnic to acknowledge the Earth's bounty and goodness. A raw food picnic is a wonderful way to celebrate this environmental holiday. An ambrosia salad is a great way to take advantage of some seasonal fruits for Earth Day, the recipe for which is in Appendix 5.

For more information visit:

http://www.earthday.org/earth-day-history-movement

http://www.huffingtonpost.com/2012/04/22/earth-day-2012-get-involved_n_1441641.html

Cinco De Mayo

Cinco De Mayo commemorates the victory of the Mexican militia over the French army at The Battle of Puebla in 1862. In the United States, Cinco De Mayo now represents a celebration of

Mexican culture, foods, and customs. Some favorite Mexican foods for the holiday include tamales and tres leches (three milk) cake, recipes for which are included in Appendix 5.

For more information visit http://www.mexonline.com/cinco -de-mayo.htm.

Summer [June 21–September 21]

On a hot summer day, there is nothing like a fresh fruit popsicle to refresh and revive! While many popsicles in the grocery store are vegan, they are also full of added sugar and preservatives. You might like to try making your own at home. Popsicle molds are inexpensive and easy to find at supermarkets, dollar stores, and other retailers during the summer. You can make popsicles as simply as pouring orange juice in the popsicle molds and freezing them, or you can go more exotic by visiting a farmer's market and finding unusual fruits. We particularly love to use fresh berries or cherries for a delicious treat. Blend them in the food processor to retain the pulp and fiber. You may need to add a little water if they are not juicy enough. Add your preferred sweetener to taste, if needed. The choice is yours, and you can be as creative as you want! We have found that adding a smidge of lemon or lime juice really enhances the flavor of our fruit popsicles. In the summer, we always have plenty of popsicles on hand for visitors; everyone always remembers the unique popsicles they enjoyed at our house!

Many people also think about churning ice cream in the summer. You are in luck if you are one of them because you *can* churn your own vegan ice cream! There are many recipes available for vegan ice cream on the internet. They use nondairy milks, some use tofu, and some use ground nuts. Some add soy creamer for texture and mouth feel. We also included a vegan ice cream cookbook in Appendix 1 called *Lick It*. In Appendix 5, we share our own recipe for a Banana Ice Cream Base. We use banana instead of adding fat for texture. This recipe is delicious as is as a banana ice cream, or you can top it with syrup, add a nut butter (such as almond), cocoa, or any number of flavors to your taste.

Summer's Seasonal Fruits and Vegetables

apricots
arugala
avocados
beets
blackberries
blueberries
boysenberries
broccoli
cabbage
cactus pears
carrots
cauliflower
celery
cherries
corn
cucumbers
dates
eggplant
figs
ginger
grapes
green beans
lemons

(Summer's Seasonal Fruits and Vegetables, Cont'd)
lettuce
melons
mulberries
nectarines
okra
olives
onions
oranges
peaches
peanuts
peas
peppers
plums
pluots
raspberries
rhubarb
spinach
strawberries
tayberries
tomatoes

July 4th

The Fourth of July, or Independence Day, celebrates the adoption of the Declaration of Independence on July 4, 1776. However, historians will tell you that the declaration was not actually signed on July 4. Regardless, July 4 is now the quintessential American holiday, celebrated with parades, fireworks, and cookouts. July 4 is usually thought of as a big meat-eating holiday with hot dogs, burgers, and ribs. While vegan hotdogs and burgers are readily available in stores, we will give you a delicious recipe for home-made vegan ribs in Appendix 5. For more information about the Fourth of July, visit

http://www.history.com/news/9-things-you-may-not-know-about-the-declaration-of-independence and

http://www.usa.gov/Topics/Independence-Day.shtml

The Feast of Mother Cabrini [Aug 24-Sept 3]

Although not a holiday per se, the Feast of Mother Cabrini is a yearly festival largely celebrated in New York. Having grown up on Long Island, I couldn't leave out such a beloved festivity with such amazing food! The feast (which is a fair, complete with rides and arcades) commemorates the life of Saint Frances Cabrini (Mother Cabrini), who spent much of her life as a missionary and founded the Missionary Sisters of the Sacred Heart. On Long Island, a yearly festival from late August to early September with carnival rides and the largest Italian feast in the area is held in Brentwood on the Suffolk Community College grounds. Among the authentic Italian cuisine enjoyed are calzones and zeppoles. In Appendix 5, we provide vegan recipes for both of these beloved treats. For those of you not familiar with zeppoles, they are a cake donut with a powdered sugar coating. Use organic powdered sugar for a superior flavor.

For more information, visit the following websites: http://www.mothercabrinifestival.org/

http://www.mothercabrini.com/legacy/life1.asp

Labor Day

Labor Day is the workingman's holiday and was first celebrated on September 5, 1882, after being organized by the New York Central Labor Union. The holiday spread geographically and became a federal holiday in 1894 to be celebrated on the first Monday of September. Parades and last summer cookouts are hallmarks of Labor Day. Since we choose for Labor Day to be a day of rest, we typically just roast Tofurky® kielbasa or brats, top with sauerkraut and/or sweet relish and/or mustard for a delicious treat. Canned vegetarian baked beans are usually also vegan; just check the label to be certain. Since Labor Day marks for many of us the official end of summer, it is also a good day to churn one more batch of ice cream.

Fall
[September 22-December 20]

Fall's Seasonal Fruits and Vegetables

apples
artichokes
arugula
Asian pears
avocados
green beans
beets
blackberries
broccoli
Brussels sprouts
burdock

(Fall's Seasonal Fruits and Vegetables, Cont'd)
cabbage
carrots
cauliflower
celery
collards
corn
cucumbers
dates
endive
fennel
figs
grapes
guavas
jicama
kale
kiwi
kumquats
leeks
lemons
lettuce
limes
Mandarin oranges
mushrooms
nectarines

(Fall's Seasonal Fruits and Vegetables, Cont'd)
okra
onions
oranges
parsnips
peaches
pears
peas
pecans
peppers
persimmons
pistachios
plums
pomegranates
potatoes
quince
raspberries
rhubarb
spinach
strawberries
sweet potatoes
turnips
walnuts

Oktoberfest

Oktoberfest is a sixteen-day festival running from late September to the first weekend of October. It was originally a celebration of the wedding of Prince Ludwig and Princess Therese who were Bavarian royalty. The citizens of Munich were invited to surrounding festivities, including a horse race that marked the end of the celebration. The horse race continued and so did Oktoberfest. Now Oktoberfest is a celebration of German, in particular Bavarian, culture with oompah bands, beer, and a variety of authentic German foods marking the occasion. Some favorites include giant soft dough pretzels, black forest cake, and liverwurst. These three recipes, made vegan, are included in Appendix 5. For more information, visit: http://www.ofest.com/history.html and http://veganfeastkitchen.blogspot.com/2012/12/vegan-liverwurst-from-world-vegan-feast.html.

Halloween

Halloween, celebrated on October 31, is derived from an ancient Celtic festival that celebrated the end of the harvest season in Gaelic culture. It was believed that on October 31, the worlds of the living and the dead overlapped, and the dead could come back to wreak havoc on the living; costumes were worn to appease the spirits. The tradition of costumes as well as that of "souling" (beggars going door to door requesting food in exchange for prayers for the souls of the dead) gave rise to the tradition of trick-or-treating. Today, candy is the mainstay of Halloween, along with popcorn balls and caramel apples. See Appendix 5 for recipes of Popcorn Balls and Gooey Caramel Apples. For more information, visit:

http://www.halloweenhistory.org/ and
http://dairyfreecooking.about.com/od/confectionscandies/r/caramelapple.htm

Thanksgiving

The first Thanksgiving was a fall harvest feast shared by the Plymouth colonists and Wampanoag Indians in 1621. Subsequent days of thanksgiving and other feasts were held regionally, but President Lincoln established the federal holiday during the Civil War in 1863. Today, the holiday is celebrated with family and friends by eating a veritable banquet of turkey, pumpkin pie, and starchy vegetable dishes. One of our favorite recipes for Thanksgiving is the stuffing I grew up with; it was made with pork sausage. We veganized it, and it is delicious! See Appendix 5 for this recipe. We also recommend you search for a vegan turkey recipe. We love the one by Alicia Simpson published in her *Vegan Celebrations* cookbook (see Appendix 1). For more information about the history of Thanksgiving, visit: http://www.history.com/topics/thanksgiving.

Winter
[December 21-March 20]

Winter's Seasonal Fruits and Vegetables

arugula
beets
blood oranges
broccoli
Brussels sprouts
cabbage
carrots
cauliflower
celery
chard
citrons
collards

(Winter's Seasonal Fruits and Vegetables, Cont'd)
endive
fava beans
fennel
guavas
jicama
kale
kiwis
leeks
lemons
lettuce
limes
Mandarin oranges
mushrooms
nettles
onions
oranges
parsnips
peanuts
pomelos
potatoes
radishes
rutabagas
spinach
winter squash
sweet potatoes
turnips

Hanukkah

Hanukkah is an eight-day celebration that commemorates the rededication of the Second Temple in Jerusalem by the Jews after they drove out their Greek-Syrian oppressors. The miracle of Hanukkah recounted in the Talmud refers to how during the rededication there was only enough candle oil to last one night, but by miracle, the oil lasted for eight nights. Today, Hanukkah is celebrated for eight nights with families gathering around the menorah to light candles and recite prayers. Each night, a candle is lit and added to the menorah for a total of eight nights with one helper candle that lights the rest. One misconception about Hanukkah is that it is the most significant Jewish holiday; that idea stems from Hanukkah's proximity to Christmas, an important Christian holiday. Hanukkah is actually a fairly minor holiday in the Jewish religion. Traditional Hanukkah dishes are typically cooked in oil (in reference to the miracle). Some of the most popular dishes are latkes (potato pancakes), kugel (a noodle casserole), and cheese blintzes. See Appendix 5 for our veganized versions of these wonderful treats. For more information, visit: http://www.history.com/topics/hanukkah.

Christmas

Christmas has been celebrated for over two thousand years as the birth date of Jesus of Nazareth, who is celebrated as the messiah in the Christian religion. December 25 is the day Christmas is celebrated; however, it is unknown what the exact day of Jesus's birth is. Early Christian leaders celebrated Christmas near the time of the pagan celebration of the winter solstice in order to increase the chances of the pagan adopting Christianity. Christmas is usually celebrated with church attendance, family gatherings, gift giving, and often with an elaborate meal including many similar dishes as Thanksgiving. One thing unique to Christmas is the baking of a wide variety of Christmas cookies. A favorite in our house is spritz cookies, a butter cookie made using a cookie press, which we share in Appendix 5. For more information about the history of Christmas, visit:

http://www.history.com/topics/christmas.

Kwanzaa

Kwanzaa, celebrated from December 26 to January 1, began during the Civil Rights movement as a means to bring the African American community together. Meaning "first fruits" in Swahili, Kwanzaa took on aspects of a variety of African harvest celebrations. Kwanzaa is a seven-night celebration in which a family gathers each night while a child lights one of the candles in the kinara (the Swahili word meaning candle-holder), and then one of the seven principles (cultural ideals) is discussed. The seven principles are unity, self-determination, collective work and responsibility, cooperative economics, purpose, creativity, and faith. There are also seven symbols of Kwanzaa: the unity cup, the kinara, mazao (harvest fruits), the mishumaa saba (seven candles representing the seven principles), the mkeka mats, the vibunzi (ear of corn), and zawadi (gifts emphasizing education and culture).

The foods enjoyed during Kwanzaa range from African recipes, to soul food, and Caribbean dishes. As for soul food, we discuss cornbread, collards, and black-eyed peas for New Years and have a recipe for regular and Buffalo Fried Chick'n for the Super Bowl. So instead of rehashing those, in Appendix 5, you will find a traditional African recipe: Peanut Soup. For more information, visit:

http://www.history.com/topics/kwanzaa-history and
http://www.sheknows.com/food-and-recipes/articles/850
319/history-of-kwanzaa-food.

New Year's Day

New Year's Day, January 1 of every year, is a time that we remember the year prior and make resolutions for the year ahead. Different countries and cultures enjoy symbolic foods on New Year's. For example, in Spain, celebrants eat twelve grapes, one at each clock stroke at midnight. Each grape represents a month in the coming year, and the flavor of the grape can signify good and bad things to come in that respective month. In the American South, our New Year's menus include collards, black-eyed peas, and cornbread symbolizing economic fortune in the New Year. The first two dishes are easy to make vegan and do not require much, if any, change. All you have to do is heat the black-eyed peas, boil the collards, and use oil or vegan butter substitute instead of any animal fat your might have used, if desired. Adding a few drops of Liquid Smoke® provides the same taste that was enjoyed when we used ham hocks. Cornbread is easy to make vegan too, but if you relied on packaged cornbread mix, you may have to change strategies. If you check the ingredients, some cornbread mixes contain animal fats and/or eggs, so it may be time to make some cornbread from scratch! See Appendix 5 for our version of homemade cornbread.

Chinese New Year

The Chinese New Year is an ancient tradition based on the traditional Chinese calendar, which was measured by lunar phases, solstices, equinoxes as well as a twelve-phase cycle comprising the Chinese zodiac. The New Year in China was traditionally a month-long celebration starting in the middle of the twelfth month and ending in the middle of the first month. Among the traditional observances were thorough cleaning of homes, ritual sacrifices of food and paper icons, and using firecrackers to scare away evil spirits. Food played a large part in celebrations; people ate fish to symbolize abundance, long noodles to symbolize long lives, and moon-shaped dumplings to symbolize family and perfection. Western influences and domestic politics forced the Chinese New Year tradition to evolve. Today the Chinese New Year is called the Spring Festival, and while it maintains some traditional aspects, the celebration focuses more on relaxation than renewing familiar ties. See Appendix 5 for our recipe for Chinese dumplings. For more information about the Chinese New Year, visit:

http://www.history.com/topics/chinese-new-year.

Super Bowl Sunday

The Super Bowl is the annual football game that determines which team will be the champion of the NFL. It is one of the biggest television events in America, with many people tuning in just to watch the big-budget commercials. Super Bowl Sunday is the second biggest day for food in America, right behind Thanksgiving. While there are plenty of snacks eaten that day, one Super Bowl favorite is buffalo chicken. While it may be hard to imagine this day ever being vegan, it is surprisingly easy! Try our Buffalo Chick'n recipe from Appendix 5. For more information on Super Bowl Sunday, visit:

http://www.fsis.usda.gov/News_&_Events/NR_012706_01/index.asp

Mardi Gras

Mardi Gras dates back thousands of years to pagan celebrations of spring and fertility. When Christianity began in Rome, religious leaders incorporated these traditions into the Christian faith to ease the transition to a new religion. Today, Mardi Gras, or Fat Tuesday, is a day of gluttony before Ash Wednesday and the beginning of Lent, which is the forty days of penance before Easter Sunday. The date of Mardi Gras varies widely from year to year. In 2013, it fell on February 12, while in 2014, it will fall on

March 4. And while Mardi Gras falls on a particular day, Mardi Gras celebrations last much longer in New Orleans! There, Mardi Gras is a raucous celebration with parades, costumes, and especially rich foods. One holiday favorite is the King Cake (named for the wise men in the Nativity story), which is a coffee cake with various nuts and fruits on the inside. On the outside, it's topped with icing and purple, yellow, and green sugars. It often has a plastic baby inside (representing the Christ child) and the person who gets the baby buys the next year's King Cake or must host the next year's party. Other good New Orleans dishes include jambalaya and beignet (pronounced bin-yay). See Appendix 5 for vegan recipes of King Cake, Jambalaya and Beignets. For more information about Mardi Gras, visit:

http://www.history.com/topics/mardi-gras,
http://www.mardigrasneworleans.com/mardi-gras-2013.html,
http://www.epicurious.com/articlesguides/holidays/mardi-gras/kingcake, and
http://www.mardigrasneworleans.com/kingcakes.html.

Valentine's Day

It is unclear which Saint Valentine (there are three) is the patron saint for the February 14th holiday. As with Mardi Gras and Ash Wednesday, St. Valentine's Day was likely timed to coincide with existing pagan fertility celebrations in Rome as a means of easing conversion. Valentine's has since become the holiday of love, with massive sales of cards, flowers, and chocolates.

It is surprisingly easy to have a vegan Valentine's Day! Chocolate is vegan unless milk or milk products are added. Many dark and semisweet chocolates are already vegan; you just need to check the labels. If you would like to make some homemade vegan treats for your sweetheart, try our recipe for Chocolate-Covered Strawberries in Appendix 5. For more information about Valentine's Day, visit: http://www.history.com/topics/valentines-day.

For all holidays, we also encourage you to check out Alicia Simpson's cookbook called *Vegan Celebrations*. It is a fabulous book that has helped bring us through many holidays for years!

SUPPLEMENTATION OR NOT?

. . . .

A question you may have about the vegan diet is whether you would need to supplement vitamins and minerals to stay healthy. You may be surprised to know that it is actually possible to follow a primarily vegan diet and not necessarily need any supplementation. A study conducted in the Tarahumara Indians of the Sierra Madre Occidental Mountains of Mexico, a population that has existed for thousands of years on a diet that is slightly greater than 95% vegan, demonstrated no significant deficiencies in either macronutrients (protein, carbohydrate and fat) or micronutrients (vitamins and minerals).[1] And even though vitamin B_{12} is found only in animal products and the Indians' intake was less than recommended by the World Health Organization (WHO), there were no deficiencies evident in this population. Apparently, the small amount of animal products they consumed, coupled with the manure used to fertilize their crops, provided enough vitamin B_{12} to sustain their health.

However, just like in the omnivore population, we as 95% vegans in America may not get all of the essential nutrients we need every day, which is why many of us routinely take vitamins to begin with.

It is definitely possible to eat a vegan diet that is *not* healthy, especially if you live off potato chips and Oreos®. Since the realities of our busy lives sometimes interfere with having the best food intake each and every day, I do recommend that my patients take a solid multivitamin/mineral supplement daily. When I say a solid multivitamin, I am referring to one that provides most, if not the entire percent daily value (% DV), which is the recommended amount you should have each day to prevent deficiencies set by the FDA, of the vitamins and minerals we may be lacking, without mega-dosing any vitamins or minerals. You can easily figure out if a vitamin/mineral supplement achieves the goal of providing most everything needed without mega-dosing just by reading the label. Under each vitamin and mineral, the label will show what % DV is contained in each tablet or capsule. If it contains much more than 100 percent, it is getting into the mega-dosing realm. As you will see, mega-dosing can cause toxic effects. On the other hand, if the supplement contains much less than 100 percent, it is not supplying enough of that component.

I will only recommend supplements that have solid science to back up their use. In Part 5, you will learn for yourself how to discern if there is good science to back up claims of dietary supplement companies. You will see that there are many supplements out there that are not supported by good science, so I recommend you not waste your money or risk your safety on these products.

Here we will discuss the micronutrients (vitamins and minerals) we require yet may be deficient in. But before we discuss specific nutrients, I would like to introduce you to the CDC's (Centers for Disease Control, a federal agency in the United States) National Health and Nutrition Examination Survey (NHANES), which is conducted by the National Center for Health Statistics (NCHS). NHANES, referred to as "N-Hanes," is a series of studies designed to collect data on the health and nutrition status of the U.S. population.[2] Blood and urine specimens are taken from a representative sample of the U.S. population for biochemical analysis of various nutrients. These measurements indicate the cumulative intake of the various nutrients, from food and supplementation sources.

In 2012, the report included fifty-eight biochemical indicators, the most comprehensive look at America's nutritional health to date. Why is it important to know about these data? Because in the end, the only thing that truly matters about any scientific health data are the health *outcomes*. Allow me to illustrate this point by using an example from the pharmaceutical industry. There is a drug called Zetia®, generic name ezetimibe, also sold in combination with a statin (simvastatin, or Zocor®) under the name Vytorin® that prevents the absorption of cholesterol, which subsequently reduces the amount of total and LDL cholesterol in the blood by around 18 percent. The logical conclusion is that this would then reduce rate of buildup of plaque responsible for heart attacks, stroke, and death. However, unlike the statin drugs, Zetia® alone does not reduce the buildup of plaque. In fact, in Merck's ENHANCE trial, a study comparing Zetia® plus simvastatin versus simvastatin alone, in the group that took Zetia® plus simvastatin, the intimal medial thickness, a measurement that serves as a marker for plaque buildup was slightly worse. In fact, no health outcomes data demonstrating reduction in heart attacks exists at all. The company withheld the information from the ENHANCE trial for two years, making billions of dollars on a drug with no known improved health outcomes![3, 4] So if a drug sold to reduce cholesterol levels does not actually reduce plaque buildup and subsequently reduce the rate of heart attacks, stroke, and death, what good is it? It is not changing the health outcomes of the people taking it. The same goes for dietary supplements. What is the point of taking supplements if they are not proven to change your health outcomes? This is how all of us should be thinking. Putting something in your body that might cause adverse consequences without even knowing there is a true benefit to be had is utterly foolish. Fortunately, when it comes to vitamins and minerals, there are well-proven health consequences when one is deficient or takes an overabundance. This is partly how the % DVs are derived.[5] That said, in the NHANES report for 2012, for most nutrition indicators, the likelihood of a demonstrated deficiency varied by age, gender, and race. For example, the elderly were more likely to be deficient in vitamin B_{12}, men were more likely to be deficient in vitamin C, and non-Hispanic Black and Mexican Americans were more likely to be deficient in vitamin D. Overall, Americans are most likely to be deficient in vitamin B_6 (10 percent), followed by iron (9.5 percent), vitamin D (8.1 percent), vitamin C (6 percent), vitamin B_{12} (2 percent), vitamin A (<1 percent), vitamin E (<1 percent), and folate (<1 percent). The study does not take into account the dietary or supplement habits of the population studied, so we can assume since most of the population are omnivores, they represented the majority of the sampling. Interestingly though, it appears that the general American population is most likely to become deficient in the nutrients most likely to be deficient in vegans: vitamin B_{12}, iron, and vitamin D.

Vitamin/Mineral Supplementation

In that we already have a handle on which vitamins and minerals are essential for good health in general, I will not provide an in-depth discussion of all of them; only the ones we are likely to become deficient in. Reading the USDA recommendations for daily intake (available at http://fnic.nal.usda.gov/dietary-guidance/dietary-reference-intakes/dri-tables) will tell you what nutrients are essential for good health and how much of each is recommended daily for healthy adults. These daily recommended intakes are based in science that has been well known for decades and is actually in excess for the average person's needs. This is to ensure adequacy for those individuals who may require more of certain nutrients to maintain good health; the recommendations should cover the vast majority of the population.

As for the vitamins themselves, it does not matter whether you get an all-natural vitamin (i.e., derived from a natural food) or one manufactured in a plant chemically. The body will use either source equally well, since the chemical structure of the individual vitamins is identical. To prove the supplement you choose to take is providing adequate quantities of the nutrients you are most likely deficient in, realize that the blood tests your doctor should draw would reflect if you were deficient in iron, vitamin B_{12}, and vitamin D, as well as other nutrients.

Vitamin B_6, also known as pyridoxine, helps to metabolize protein, maintain the nervous system and the immune system and is instrumental in the formation of hemoglobin (the part of the red blood cell that carries oxygen).[6] It may also help prevent cardiovascular disease by reducing homocysteine levels. People most prone to vitamin B_6 deficiency are those with impaired renal function, autoimmune disorders, and those with alcohol dependence. Deficiency in infants has been known to cause seizures.[7] Adult symptoms of deficiency include cracks at the lips and gums, tongue enlargement, anemia, numbness and tingling in the arms and legs, muscle cramps, respiratory infections, birth defects, hair loss, and eczema. Vitamin B_6 is available in fish, organ meats, starchy vegetables (such as potatoes), and fruit (except citrus). However, since vitamin B_6 deficiency has even been noted in people who take supplements, but higher rates are reported for those who do not take supplements, I highly recommend you take a supplement that has 100 percent of the daily value, on top of your healthy vegan diet.

Adequate iron intake is necessary for our bodies to synthesize healthy amounts of hemoglobin and myoglobin.[8] As noted previously, hemoglobin transports oxygen to other cells in the body. Myoglobin is a protein found in muscle tissue. Inadequate iron intake facilitates the development of iron deficiency anemia. It is important to remember that iron is a heavy metal; excessive intake can lead to iron poisoning. Severe iron poisoning can lead to coma and death.[9]

In Part 2, we discussed the concerns about adults who do not consume adequate amounts of vitamin D. Vitamin D is a fat-soluble vitamin that is naturally present in very few foods, other than the ones intentionally fortified with it. Our bodies produce it when the UV rays from the sun strike the skin and trigger its synthesis. However, it is clear from the NHANES data that we are not producing enough vitamin D to prevent a deficiency. Since your vitamin D blood level is easy enough for your physician to obtain, I recommend you start there in terms of deciding how much vitamin D you need to supplement. On the one hand, vitamin D deficiency has been associated with several chronic conditions and their degree of severity, so you want to ensure your vitamin D intake is adequate. On the other hand, vitamin D being a fat-soluble vitamin, it can be stored in the body if taken in excess. This can lead to excessively high blood levels of calcium, which can cause nausea, constipation, heart arrhythmias, and kidney stones. However, since vitamin D deficiency is much more likely than vitamin D toxicity, I prefer to err on the side of ensuring I get adequate amounts and let my blood work tell me how I am doing. In my personal experience, I not only take a multivitamin with 100 percent the RDA of vitamin D, I also take a calcium tablet with vitamin D and two vitamin D capsules containing 400 IU vitamin D, just to maintain my blood levels in the mid-normal range. Please work with your physician to figure out what is best for you.

Vitamin C, also known as ascorbic acid, is required for the growth and repair of body tissues. It aids in wound healing and plays a key role in repairing cartilage, bones, and teeth. It also aids in the absorption of iron from the GI tract through its ability to cause reduction. Vitamin C is also a potent antioxidant, which we will discuss separately. It is widely available in fruits, especially citrus, and vegetables such as broccoli, Brussels sprouts, spinach, winter squash, and green and red peppers.[10] The disease known as scurvy results from severe vitamin C deficiency. Scurvy was reported as early as the Middle Ages and was common to sailors from the fifteenth to the nineteenth century as technology allowed them to stay longer at sea without fresh fruits and vegetables. It starts out with fatigue and then swelling gums that easily bleed upon touch.[11] The gums ultimately rot, giving off a putrid odor. Eventually, the skin itself hemorrhages easily; ulcers form and become gangrenous. Death results presumably from hemorrhaging in the brain and heart. The good news is that even in the later stages of scurvy, high doses of vitamin C can cure the patient. Those most likely to suffer from vitamin C deficiency today are smokers and passive smokers (those inhaling second-hand smoke), people with chronic kidney disease, severe malabsorption syndromes, and cancer patients.

Vitamin C has been studied for benefits in preventing various health issues, such as cardiovascular disease, cancer, and the common cold. A review of studies in the Cochrane database from 1966 to 2006 revealed that in studies in which a minimum of 200 mg per day of vitamin C were taken prophylactically, the incidence of colds did not decrease in the average person.[12] (The Cochrane database reviews are internationally recognized as the highest standard in evidence-based medicine.) However, there were moderate reductions in the *duration* of colds (8 percent in adults). No significant differences from placebo were seen in those who began taking large doses of vitamin C after a cold started. Interestingly, marathon runners, skiers, and soldiers in subarctic exercises who took large amounts of vitamin C prophylactically did have a 50 percent reduction in the *incidence* of colds.

While the role of vitamin C and cancer has been widely discussed, there is a lack of evidence supporting its use orally as an adjunct cancer treatment. More recently, studies using vitamin C administered intravenously (IV) have been proposed since giving vitamin C by IV may allow for more pharmaceutical and therefore therapeutic levels to help kill cancer cells. Since these pharmaceutical levels kill cancer cells in vitro (i.e., a test tube environment), scientists proposed relooking at whether intravenous vitamin C can improve outcomes in cancer patients.[13] However, in a Phase I clinical study of patients with advanced malignancies previously treated, 4 doses of vitamin C up to 1,500 mg/kg body weight three times per week failed to demonstrate any clinical benefit.[14]

Since the body cannot store excess amounts of vitamin C, excessive chronic dosing of vitamin C is not usually thought to create serious adverse health consequences.[15] However, some have theorized that excess vitamin C intake may cause kidney stones, and this theory appears to be relevant in people who take 1–2 grams per day, which is seventeen to thirty-three times the amount of the recommended daily intake.[16, 17]

Other symptoms a person taking high doses of vitamin C may experience include diarrhea, nausea, and abdominal cramps.

Vitamin B_{12}, also known as cyanocobalamine, is essential for nerve functioning as well as red blood cell and DNA formation.[18] A deficiency in vitamin B_{12} is evident when the CBC reveals the presence of megaloblastic anemia. This means that the red blood cells themselves are unusually large because they cannot divide due to inhibition of DNA synthesis. The MCV (mean cell volume) measurement, which is part of the CBC, tells us how large the red blood cells are. Clinical signs and symptoms, such as fatigue and pale skin, coupled with low levels of vitamin B_{12} in the blood would confirm if you are deficient. In addition, Vitamin B_{12} requires a substance known as *intrinsic factor*, which is present in our GI tracts, to be absorbed into the blood stream and used by the body. As we get older, we produce less and less intrinsic factor, which may require either a higher dose of oral vitamin B_{12} or, in more severe cases, vitamin B_{12} injections. (Whether you are vegan or not has no effect on intrinsic factor.) Vitamin B_{12} deficiency due to inadequate intrinsic factor is called pernicious anemia.

Vitamin B_{12} is found in animal products such as meat, eggs, and dairy. It is also sometimes found in cereals that have been intentionally fortified with vitamin B_{12}. As a 95% vegan, it is possible you will still receive enough vitamin B_{12} to prevent a deficiency. However, to be on the safe side, I recommend anyone following a plant-based diet take a vitamin B_{12} supplement. Most commercially available multivitamin supplements contain 100 percent the recommended daily intake of vitamin B_{12}. In addition, since vitamin B_{12} is a water-soluble vitamin, meaning that whatever your body doesn't need it will eliminate through the urine, it is generally okay to take up to twice as much of the percent daily value without any problems, if you find you need it as an older adult. You can buy vitamin B_{12} by itself and take in addition to your solid multivitamin. Of course, your doctor can also tell you if he doesn't think your vitamin B_{12} intake is adequate through your CBC and other measurements before you go to the trouble and expense of taking more than the daily requirement.

Vitamin A, also known as retinol, helps to form and maintain healthy bone and soft tissue, as well as a healthy immune system. It also promotes better vision, particularly in low light.[19] The biologically active form of vitamin A comes from animal sources, meat, and dairy. Beta-carotene is a *provitamin* of vitamin A; it must be converted to the active form of vitamin A in our bodies. Beta-carotene is widely present in bright-yellow and orange fruits and vegetables, such as carrots, sweet potatoes, pumpkin, apricots, and winter squash. The general rule is that the deeper the color of these vegetables, the higher the beta-carotene content is. Beta-carotene is also present in green vegetables, such as green leafy vegetables as well as broccoli. Deficiency of vitamin A manifests itself as night blindness and corneal lesions in the eye. The deficiency can be confirmed through a blood test for serum retinol.[20] Since vitamin A is a fat soluble vitamin, excess amounts are stored in the liver. Thus, excess amounts of vitamin A can become toxic. However, note that excessive amounts of beta-carotene are not toxic but can cause the skin to turn orange, which is not dangerous, only strange-looking. Acute vitamin A toxicity is caused by taking several hundred thousands IUs (international units) at one time; whereas, chronic toxicity occurs from taking doses higher than recommended over a period. Both can have serious consequences, including death. Typical symptoms of vitamin A toxicity include dizziness, headache, dry, scaly skin, liver tenderness, double vision, joint pains, and hemorrhages.[21] It can also cause birth defects. The vegan diet can provide plenty of beta-carotene to meet the nutritional needs for vitamin A, provided enough fruits and vegetables are consumed. But again, to be on the safe side, you can choose to supplement your diet with a solid multivitamin to ensure you are getting enough. Taking one solid multivitamin per day on top of your healthy vegan diet will not create toxicity in healthy adults.

Vitamin E is a collective name for several fat-soluble compounds called tocopherols. It has many different bodily functions, including maintaining immune function and gene expression.[22] It is also an antioxidant; it stops the production of free radicals. We will discuss antioxidants separately below. Vitamin E is found in nuts, seeds, and vegetable oils. Deficiency symptoms include lowered immune function, numbness tingling, and pain in the extremities, muscle weakness, and retinal degeneration leading to blindness.

Although vitamin E *supplements* have been touted to prevent heart disease, the clinical studies conducted to look objectively at the issue have not proven this theory.[23, 24, 25, 26, 27, 28, 29] On the other hand, a large study conducted in Finland demonstrated that higher intakes of vitamin E from *food sources* were associated with reduced death from coronary heart disease in both men and women.[30] However, it has been postulated that the studies with the vitamin E *supplements* were conducted in older patients; perhaps if the vitamin E supplements were studied over a longer period in younger patients, the outcomes might be different.

The role of vitamin E in the prevention of cancer has also been explored extensively. Unfortunately, vitamin E has not been shown to be beneficial in general. For example, in a large clinical trial involving over thirty-five thousand men, vitamin E supplementation did not show any benefit over placebo in the prevention of prostate cancer.[31] And although there have been other studies to indicate the benefit of vitamin E in preventing cancer[32], those studies could not be replicated.[33]

Vitamin E supplements do have the potential to interact with certain medications, as well as become stored in excess in the liver, so I do not recommend taking more than 100% of the DV. Vitamin E can inhibit platelet aggregation, which can potentiate the effects of other anticoagulants, which can lead to bleeding and hemorrhage. It can also reduce the effectiveness of chemotherapy agents by protecting cancer cells through its antioxidant effect.

Also, you should know that in a large meta-analysis of nineteen randomized trials, a dose-dependent relationship between the dose of vitamin E and all cause mortality was observed.[34] The higher the dose of vitamin E, the higher the death rate from all possible causes. Of course, as we have discussed, this doesn't mean that vitamin E *causes* death; however in large doses, there appears to be a *correlation*. The theory behind this observation is that in high doses, vitamin E demonstrates pro-oxidant properties. This means that it would act contrary to its usual antioxidant actions. Patients who already had chronic disease in this study seemed to be particularly susceptible to the hazards of excessive vitamin E supplementation.

Folate (also known as folic acid in its non-salt form) is a water-soluble B vitamin. It is widely available in bean and legumes, citrus fruits, green leafy vegetables, and whole grains. Deficiency of folate manifests itself as a megaloblastic anemia, which may cause excessive fatigue. Mouth sores, gray hair, poor growth, and birth defects can also occur from folate deficiency. Folate deficiency can occur due to alcohol abuse, digestive diseases such as celiac and Crohn's, interactions with medications such as phenytoin and sulfa antibiotics, and eating overcooked food.[35] A folate deficiency can be diagnosed through your CBC and other blood tests. Since folate is water-soluble, it does not accumulate when consumed in excessive quantities so is not generally thought to become toxic.

The NHANES report did not include any biomarkers to indicate if Americans are receiving sufficient calcium or other mineral intake. Green leafy vegetables, such as spinach, kale, and collard greens, can supply quite a bit of calcium in the vegan diet. Likewise, if using calcium-fortified soy or other nondairy milk, you will receive a healthy dose of calcium there as well. Some multivitamins contain more calcium than they have in the past, so you may not need to go to the extra expense of buying a separate calcium source. Your physician can tell you if he or she feels you need to supplement your diet with additional calcium. Keep in mind that calcium is optimally absorbed in the presence of adequate vitamin D, so if you do take a calcium supplement, take it with one that also contains vitamin D.

As for other minerals, such as zinc, magnesium, and iodine, your solid multivitamin/mineral supplement should provide plenty for good health.

Again, a safe solution to prevent vitamin/mineral deficiencies for all of us is to start by taking a solid multivitamin supplement daily that supplies all of the essential nutrients any of us, vegan or not, could miss in a day. Because there are essential nutrients in which the recommended daily intake is different for adult men versus adult women, as well as age differences, you will find that many vitamin/mineral supplements are labeled for men and women at different life stages. For example women, particularly if they are still menstruating or menstruate heavily, may require up to twice as much iron daily as men. Based on all of the available data, it would not be wise to take a vitamin/mineral supplement that contains more than 100 percent of the DV for any individual component, unless directed by your physician. Please be sure to read the labels, and choose wisely.

The Role of Antioxidants

Given the level of interest in antioxidants, along with the fact that we receive most of our antioxidants through food consumption, we should discuss them more at length. While certain vitamins have been identified as having antioxidant properties, there are potentially thousands more chemicals that are not isolated in supplements, and only available in the fruits and vegetables we eat. These are most often referred to as flavonoids and phytochemicals. Following a healthy 95% vegan diet will supply a wide variety of these antioxidants, much more so than the typical American diet.

Antioxidants are substances that bind to and rid the body of free radicals. Free radicals are highly reactive forms of oxygen or nitrogen. They have an unpaired electron in the outer orbit, which causes to them to quickly bind to any nearby substances that offer to stabilize them. In turn, these other molecules can then become free radicals, setting off a whole chain of reactions that can ultimately damage bodily proteins, including DNA.

Free radicals are actually generated in our bodies daily through various biochemical processes. Oddly enough, they do play an important role in helping us fight off pathogens such as viruses, bacteria, and fungi, but in excess quantities, they can create significant health issues. While nature provides each of our cells the ability to fight off the free radicals normally present from our biochemical processes, this system of balancing can become overwhelmed in the face of exposure to more free radicals generated due to environmental contamination.

Exposure to environmental pollutants including cigarette smoke, radiation, UV light, and various chemicals such as pesticides increases the amount of free radicals our bodies must fight off. *Oxidative stress* is the term for what occurs when we are unable to fight off all of the free radical exposure, and it has been implicated in over one hundred diseases, as well as contributing greatly to the aging process.[36] In fact, oxidative stress has been shown to induce tissue injury implicated in cardiovascular disease, cancer, rheumatoid arthritis, Alzheimer's disease, Parkinson's disease, and complications of diabetes such as retinopathy and peripheral nerve damage.

Well-known antioxidants include vitamin C, vitamin E, and vitamin A. Both selenium and zinc are minerals that also act as antioxidants. But just as you start to think, *maybe I should just take more of those vitamins and minerals,* let me remind you there are no consistent data showing this strategy is beneficial. In fact, in one double-blind, placebo controlled study of over eighteen thousand smokers, former smokers, and workers exposed to asbestos in which 30 mg beta-carotene and 25,000 IU of retinol were given, after four years of follow-up there was not only no benefit in the treatment group, the supplementation may actually have had an adverse effects on the incidence and risk of death from lung cancer.[37] In fact, the balance of various antioxidants provided by nature in the fruits and vegetables we consume appear to be our best defense against free radicals.[38] This may be due to the fact that different antioxidants work in different ways. Some of them stop oxidation before it starts, some scavenge free radicals, and some stabilize the chain reaction. Thus, taking more of one type of antioxidant is not productive because all of the various antioxidants need to balance and work in concert with each other. Supplementing one type of antioxidant is like trying to make an orchestra out of one instrument. You can have sixty drummers, but that's not what you need for an orchestra; you need violins, trumpets, and a variety of other instruments all working together to have a symphony.

Thus, the potent protective properties of the vegan diet are likely in the additive and synergistic effects of the complex phytochemicals in fruit and vegetables.[39] There are a variety of natural chemicals found in fruits and vegetables that have also been identified as having antioxidant properties, but they are not all available in supplement form.

In fact, there is no supplement on the market that can mimic what nature provides us.

This is why it is so important to consume a wide variety of fresh (or frozen) whole foods; you would not otherwise take in these other wonderful antioxidants.

One of the best parts of following a vegan diet is the fact that by consuming a wide variety of fruits and vegetables, you will be increasing your intake of antioxidants. When you see all of the colors in fruits, reds, oranges, yellows, blues, and purples, think *antioxidants*. The same goes for all of the colors in the various vegetables. Many herbs, spices and teas contain an abundance of antioxidants. Food from nature is simply an endless source of great nutrition!

Now I would like to turn our attention to a specific antioxidant that has gained much attention in the last few years. Although it first became widely known in 1959,[40] Coenzyme Q has only been intensively studied for health outcomes in the last twenty years. Coenzyme Q is a group of naturally occurring, fat-soluble compounds called lipoquinones. Although it is present in all human cells (it is also called ubiquinone for that reason), it is present in the highest quantities in the mitochondria (often called "the powerhouse of the cell") of heart tissue in animals. In nature, it is also present in smaller quantities in the roots and leaves of plants. It is a free radical scavenger and assists the heart mitochondria in converting the energy in carbohydrates and fatty acids into ATP, the energy source utilized by the muscle tissue. Our bodies naturally make Coenzyme Q but in smaller quantities as we get older. Also, the statins, used to lower LDL cholesterol levels interfere with our natural production of Coenzyme Q.

Knowing all of this, a logical next thought would be, "Since it is present in our heart and aids in energy production for the heart, wouldn't it help to take a Coenzyme Q supplement? Wouldn't it be good for my heart?" and "If we produce lesser quantities as we get older and statins inhibit our bodies from making it, should we begin to supplement it as we get older and in people who take statins?" and "If the heart needs energy to beat and contract, would people with heart failure benefit from taking a Coenzyme Q supplement?"

There have been so many studies published looking at various parameters of Coenzyme Q's effects in humans; it is impossible to discuss all of them here. However, the bottom line is that the studies conducted to date have been in small numbers of patients, and the results have been highly variable, which is why Coenzyme Q is not routinely recommended within the medical community or in the American Heart Association's various guidelines for the management of cardiac patients. Some of the studies also did not have sufficient controls in place, so the conclusions are not considered to be credible in the scientific community.

That said, it is also important to note that different studies used different dosages of Coenzyme Q, with the lower doses usually not showing any benefit. The studies were also over different lengths of time as well, which is an important consideration in looking at any potential benefit in treating or preventing chronic disease. It takes time to really judge what the health outcomes in humans will be. For example, in a small study in which thirty patients with congestive heart failure were randomized to a double-blind crossover trial to either 100 mg of Coenzyme Q or placebo for three months (see chapter on "Becoming Your Own Scientist" for further information on how to evaluate the value of clinical trials), Coenzyme Q failed to improve left ventricular functionality (the left ventricle has to pump hard because the blood that comes out of it then goes to the rest of the body) or quality of life.[41] However, in a study in which 319 patients with congestive heart failure were studied in a randomized, double-blind fashion over period of a year, Coenzyme Q (versus placebo) significantly reduced hospitalizations for the worsening of heart failure as well as the incidence of pulmonary edema (fluid in the lungs) and cardiac asthma. The dose used in this study was 2 mg/kg body weight, which equates to 136 mg in a patient weighing 150 lb.[42] In another study in which 121 patients were randomized to receive either Coenzyme Q 300 mg or placebo for two weeks prior to elective coronary bypass surgery, those taking Coenzyme Q demonstrated a quicker recovery of cardiac contractility (the heart muscle's force of contraction) following the surgery. The Coenzyme Q group also required fewer drugs to help the heart contract than did the placebo patients, but the study was not powered such that this difference could be stated as significantly different.[43] And in a smaller study in which twenty-three patients with chronic heart failure were randomized to either Coenzyme Q 100 mg three times daily (for a total of 300mg per day) or placebo for four weeks in a double-blind cross-over fashion, patients taking Coenzyme Q had improved functional capacity with respect to exercise training.[44]

In patients who take statins to control their cholesterol level, there appears to be a dose-related decline in circulating Coenzyme Q levels; the higher the dose of the statin, the more depleted in Coenzyme Q the person becomes.[45] At the same time, many patients report muscle pain while taking statins. Researchers believe the muscle pain is tied to Coenzyme Q depletion. Several small studies have been conducted to determine if Coenzyme Q supplementation would help relieve muscle pain, with conflicting results.[46] And although in several small studies Coenzyme Q has demonstrated a reduction in muscle pain, a large, well-controlled study is needed to *conclusively prove* that Coenzyme Q can alleviate the muscle pain associated with statin treatment.

Another potential effect of Coenzyme Q in its capacity as an antioxidant is that it can help preserve nitric oxide. Nitric oxide relaxes peripheral arteries, which in turn lowers blood pressure.[47] While some studies have shown a benefit of reducing blood pressure with Coenzyme Q, some have not. Again, the dosages used do seem to make a difference. The reductions in blood pressure are mild but may be enough to complement other blood pressure medication to help you reach your target. It is *very* important that you not stop taking your blood pressure medicine without consulting your physician. Keep in mind that while Coenzyme Q *may* reduce your blood pressure, it may not reduce it enough to reach the target you need to prevent the complications of hypertension, such as heart attack, stroke, kidney disease, and blindness.

The problem with all of the claimed potential benefits of Coenzyme Q from the perspective of the scientific medical community is that none of the small studies showing a benefit to taking it have been replicated in larger and longer well-controlled studies demonstrating true patient outcomes that would instill confidence that the smaller studies' conclusions are valid. Likewise, there are also many small studies in which Coenzyme Q did not show a benefit in various parameters, but these too have never been replicated in a larger study. Why? Larger studies are extremely expensive—in the millions of dollars. Who would fund such a study? Certainly not drug companies; they make money on their drugs and have no incentive to compare their drugs to Coenzyme Q. What about the companies that manufacture and distribute Coenzyme Q? They are not required to do so by the FDA, so why would they invest that kind of money when they can sit back and make plenty of money without the studies? Yet highly recognized and competent medical groups will not recommend Coenzyme Q without solid, irrefutable data. This is where the supplement/nutriceutical industry needs to step up to the plate and invest in the proper studies to support their claims. Let's see if that happens; I am not optimistic as long as the FDA does not mandate it.

So for now, with Coenzyme Q, only you can decide if you would like to spend the money on a yet "unproven" supplement. Since there are relatively few side effects associated with Coenzyme Q supplementation, you may wish to give it a try if you have hypertension, suffer from muscle pain from statins, or have heart failure. My only recommendations are that if you are going to take Coenzyme Q, take an adequate dose (200–300 mg per day), and if you are allergic to it, do not take it. Also, be aware that Coenzyme Q can interact with some medications. For example, it can increase the risk of bleeding in patients taking antiplatelet drugs such as aspirin or Plavix®.[48] On the flip side, it can inhibit the action of Coumadin® (also known as warfarin), counteracting its anticoagulant effect.[47] Because it may have an additive effect to blood pressure medicine, it is possible your blood pressure may go lower than your target.[49] Coenzyme Q can also improve the beta-cell activity of the pancreas, enhancing insulin activity.[50] In patients taking sulfonylureas (such as glipizide or glyburide) or insulin, it can cause the blood sugar to go too low (less than 70 mg/dl).[51]

In summary, I hope you can see why questions about whether you should take a supplement that has no daily requirement for life can be a very complex one to answer. In the case of Coenzyme Q, it may help, and it is unlikely to hurt unless there is a significant drug interaction or you are allergic to it. If you are having muscle pain with a statin and there are no contraindications for you to try Coenzyme Q, it may be worth a try. It would be far better to try this supplement than to stop taking your statin. Likewise, if you are unable to reach the target goal for your blood pressure, you may wish to discuss trying Coenzyme Q with your physician. The same goes for heart failure patients. I discussed Coenzyme Q specifically to begin to show you the research and thought process that should go behind a decision to put a substance into your body. In the section "Becoming Your Own Scientist," we will discuss further how you can begin to do this research for yourself. I hope you will become very discerning when it comes to putting anything into your body, and as always, consult your physician with any questions.

EXERCISE AND SLEEP

· ·

When you first decided to read this book, you were most likely excited to learn more about following a healthy vegan diet. But the truth is, good nutrition is just one piece of the good health picture. Good nutrition needs to be balanced with healthy doses of exercise and sleep, not smoking, and efforts to control blood pressure, cholesterol levels, and blood glucose with the use of medications, if needed.

Exercise can assist greatly in your efforts to control your blood pressure, manage your lipid levels, and manage your mood. Exercise accompanied by weight loss can also reduce levels of C-reactive protein (CRP), a marker of internal inflammation associated with cardiovascular events.[1] Reduced levels of CRP likely occur as a secondary benefit of exercise reducing body fat.[2] Also, a meta-analysis of randomized, controlled clinical studies demonstrated that aerobic exercise reduced blood pressure in people with high blood pressure *and* normal blood pressure, in both overweight *and* lean study subjects.[3] In another meta-analysis, both aerobic exercise and resistance training was also shown to reduce blood pressure in patients with hypertension.[4] Lipid levels have been shown to be favorably affected by exercise. Specifically, HDL (the good cholesterol) levels increase with exercise, and it appears that the number of exercise sessions, rather than exercise intensity, has more of an impact on HDL.[5] The American Diabetes Association recommends 150 minutes of exercise each week, with no more than two days passing between exercise activities.[6] This 150 minutes can be achieved in any number of ways: 30 minutes a day for 5 days in a week, 45 minutes twice, then 1 hour on another day, or even 15 minutes at a time.

What type of exercise should you do? Based on the literature cited above, pretty much anything that moves your body more than your body moves now will be beneficial. This is great news; you don't have to become an aerobics queen or body builder for exercise to improve your health status! I would advise you to discuss what may be best for you with your physician. He or she knows your physical condition best. Importantly, choose something you can stick with for the long haul. I get bored easily, so I mix it up to ensure I can stick to my goal of 150 minutes or more per week. For example, one day, I may walk my dog for 45 minutes, and come home and lift weights for another 15 minutes. For the next session, I may go to the gym and exercise on the elliptical for 30 minutes, then lift weights with my personal trainer for another 30 minutes. Then I may go to a yoga or Pilates class at the next session. Some weeks I may not get all 150 minutes in, so I may get more than 150 minutes the next week. Some weeks I just want to do yoga, other weeks I may even jog. The point is, I do the best I can. I am certainly not perfect, but what I am doing is clearly working for me, based on my weight, my blood work, and my blood pressure. Truthfully, sometimes it is difficult to get myself to the gym or outside to walk or jog. As I said, I am not perfect. However, I have found that reminding myself that I am never *sorry* I went and always feel great afterward almost always gets me out the door.

There are other reasons it is important to exercise on top of influencing metabolic parameters. Exercise helps people with arthritis to maintain their functionality and range of motion.[7] If exercise can help people who have rheumatoid arthritis, it stands to reason it can help the rest of us maintain our functionality and range of motion. If you live a longer life but have lost your ability to climb stairs, walk through a theme park with your grandchildren, and other activities that require you to keep up with the people you love, then what is the point?

If you cannot afford to have a gym membership (or just don't like the gym), perhaps working out at home would work for you. There exists many, many wonderful exercise DVDs out there. If you have Netflix® or some other streaming video service, search through all of the exercise programs. There are programs for just stretching, for yoga, for aerobics, for dancing, and for strength training out there. If you cannot afford exercise equipment, use what you do have: furniture, cans of food, bags of kitty litter, and any other creative ideas you may have. The more exercise you do, the more you will come to depend on how wonderful it makes you feel, not to mention the positive changes you will see in your blood work!

One important thing to note about exercise versus appetite and food intake: it is very easy to out-eat the calorie burning benefits of exercise. For example, a thirty-minute walk burns around 100 calories. Sitting down and drinking a regular beer afterward adds 150 calories, more than you burned walking. Jogging for forty-five minutes might burn around 400 calories. But taking the attitude that you can eat whatever you want because you ran forty-five minutes is dangerous. Eating just 400 calories more will undo the great work you have done by exercising. We have all seen people who say they work out routinely, but they still have a spare tire around the middle. The reason is simple: they are not disciplining themselves on the food front. Just be aware of this tendency so that you don't get caught out-eating your exercise efforts.

Few people think of sleep as being a piece of their physical health, which is why I wanted to address it in this book. In fact, sleep deprivation can affect your metabolic and cardiovascular health.[8] It is not just daytime drowsiness you suffer when you lose sleep.

Through various mechanisms, sleep deprivation can lead or contribute to hypertension. Through various hormonal changes that occur in sleep deprivation, appetite naturally increases. Also, normal glucose metabolism is altered to the point of potentiating insulin resistance. The size and number of fat cells increases. Ultimately, the internal storm that is occurring potentiates inflammatory processes and increases the risk of diabetes, cardiovascular disease, immune dysfunction, and mortality.

Sleep apnea is a specific sleep disorder in which the person's breathing is interrupted, sometimes hundreds of times during the night. *Obstructive sleep apnea* occurs when there is an anatomical blockage in the airway, preventing the free flow of breathing. It can occur in people who are overweight or obese and those who have other anatomical aberrations, such as a deviated septum, large tonsils, a big tongue, or a large neck. *Central sleep apnea* occurs when the brain fails to signal the breathing muscles to breathe. Sleep apnea is a serious medical condition. It can lead to the consequences of sleep deprivation we discussed previously, as well as worsening of psychological issues, such as depression and ADHD.

If you have been told you stop breathing or gasp frequently when you sleep, it is important for you to discuss this with your physician. Your physician may recommend you have a sleep study in order to identify the potential cause(s). There are different treatment options to correct sleep apnea, depending on the identified cause. Losing weight can also help to resolve sleep apnea.

Not every reason for sleep deprivation can be cured. For example, being up frequently in the night for a newborn infant is a reality you can't change until the baby sleeps through the night. Without any obvious causes for sleep deprivation, you should discuss the issue with your physician. The solution can be as simple as not watching TV for a couple of hours before retiring or as complex as having surgery to correct and anatomical condition. Whatever the case, knowing that your lack of sleep can actually set you up for an increased risk of serious health problems, I hope you will address any sleep issues you may have.

PART 4:
Strategies for Specific Medical Issues

WEIGHT LOSS

∙ ∙

According to the CDC (Centers for Disease Control) statistics, in just ten years, from 2000 to 2010, the United States went from having no states having an obesity prevalence of 30 percent to twelve states having a 30 percent prevalence of obesity. In addition, no state has met the Healthy People 2010 goal of reducing the prevalence of obesity to 15 percent (see http://www.cdc. gov/obesity/data/adult.html). As of the writing of this book, 35.7 percent of the U.S. population is obese (recall that obesity is defined as a BMI of 30 or greater, and a BMI of 25–29 is considered overweight). Presently, 33.3 percent of American adults are overweight (see http://www.cdc.gov/nchs/fastats/overwt.htm). This means that in total, 66 percent of all American adults are overweight or obese!

At the same time, the rates of diabetes, heart disease, and cancer related to obesity have climbed significantly. Cancers associated with obesity include breast, uterus, colon, esophagus, pancreatic, kidney, and prostate. Besides diabetes and heart disease, people who are obese are much more prone to blood clots in the lungs and legs, sleep apnea, stroke, pancreatitis, infertility, arthritis, and gout. If ever there was a good reason to lose weight, pick any one of these ailments—none of them are any fun! To protect our children and future generations from the ravages of obesity, we must include them in our healthy decisions; we must create a ripple effect. It would be even better if, with future generations, we just prevented obesity from the start by teaching them good nutrition practices.

If all you ate were raw, whole foods (legumes, whole grains, fruits, and vegetables) with no added fat, you likely would not need a structured meal plan. You would not have insulin surges that make you hungrier later in the day, and you would receive adequate nutrition. It would be very easy to lose weight for the vast majority of readers, if all they ate were whole foods. If you can live in that way, great! You do not need to read the rest of this chapter. However, if you want meals that require recipes and want the ability to fit in at social dining situations, this chapter will help you. It is easy to overeat when a hot meal is on the table. If you love cookies, pies, cakes, and other desserts, this chapter will explain how you can fit these items into a healthy weight loss plan. This chapter will empower you and give you tools to control your food intake.

How many weight loss diets have you tried? There are dozens of them out there, and they will all create weight loss by one simple strategy: they provide fewer calories per day than the number of calories it takes to maintain your body weight. That's it. As we saw in Part 1, even a low-carb diet creates weight loss in that way; it just creates a greater weight loss in the beginning because the dieter loses more water in the beginning.

In my experience, something will work for every person. You just need to find the right diet to work best with your psyche and lifestyle. Many people have lost weight and kept it off with Weight Watchers®. Then there are the various programs that supply prepackaged food. Then there are the fad diets that do not provide appropriate nutrition. Fad diets tend to be easier to follow initially because they focus on what to eat and when to eat. However, they tend to cut calories so low and eliminate favorite foods such that that no one can follow them for very long, and people don't know what to do when they have finished the fad diet to maintain the weight loss. Here I will provide the tools you need to construct a *customized for you* healthy vegan weight loss program, with a few familiar options to implement it. You can choose whatever will work best for your psyche and lifestyle. You may choose to do the following:

1. Count calories.

2. Use the 95% Vegan Food Choices™ Plan.

3. Use the 95% Vegan BUC™ Plan.

4. Develop your own plan based on the guidance provided in this chapter.

Any of these will work for you once you identify the appropriate calorie level to lose and maintain your new weight. Also, you can switch from one method to another at any time.

To begin, let me share a little secret with you. If you can identify the appropriate calorie level to maintain the weight you want to achieve, that is a great calorie level to lose and then maintain that weight. This is because from the start, you know what you will have to do to maintain that weight, so by following a plan with that amount of calories from the beginning, you will truly begin the lifestyle habits you need for your lifetime to remain at that healthier weight, with a healthier diet. Fad diets that cut calories to 1,200 or below to create a quick weight loss leave you dangling; you have not identified the best way to maintain that weight loss. In addition, you have been starving yourself to the point of being ravenously hungry, so it is easy to slip and regain all of the weight and more.

The second secret I would like to share with you is that never in my career have I ever put anyone on 1,200 calories or below to lose weight. The minimum is 1,400 calories, and this is generally for shorter, older women. The taller you are, the younger you are, the more exercise you get all dictate being able to eat more calories to lose and maintain your weight. The plan we devise for you here is going to be doable for the long haul. As you will see, I include a dessert for every calorie level. There are no foods you will have to cut out, just the excess portions which are maintaining your current weight.

The 95% Vegan Food Choices™ Plan for each calorie level ensures an adequate intake of protein, the amino acid lysine in particular, since the requirements for other essential amino acids are easily covered within the food choices. Each calorie level also allows for less than 30 percent of calories coming from fat, which is in line with American Heart Association guidelines (see http://circ.ahajournals.org/content/119/8/1161). If you can cut out even more fat, that is great. If not, at least you know you are within the guidelines established by a highly credible organization.

Each list for the 95% Vegan Food Choices™ Plan will indicate how many calories, grams of protein, fat, fiber, and carbohydrate are in each choice on the list. This will help you when you prepare vegan cookbook recipes in that you will be able to approximate how many servings of each choice are in a serving of the recipe. Just consider where the major ingredients fall. For example, if the largest ingredient is some type of bean, then you know you will be counting a portion of legumes. Does it have enough vegetable or fruit in it to count for a serving or two? If so, you will count one or both of those lists. Once you have your major lists taken care of in terms of number of servings of legumes, grains, fruits, and vegetables, if the servings don't account for the amount of fat in the recipe, determine how many grams of fat remain. How much of a portion does the remaining fat in the recipe call for? We will go through an example of this toward the end of this chapter.

The 95% Vegan BUC™ Plan is another way to ensure you are within the calorie allowance for your plan. BUC stands for "Because U(you) Can," meaning you have the flexibility to follow a point-oriented system to lose weight. By using the BUC Plan but also ensuring you are getting around the same amount of protein, fruits, and vegetables similar to that of the choices plan, you will count to a much lower number each day. Many people find that easier than actually counting calories into quadruple digits. However, if you prefer to count calories, you have that as yet another option.

As you follow your plan and get better at becoming vegan, it will become easier and easier. You just need to continue trying each day to get better. If you falter, get right back on it the next day. Do not let The Guilt Factor (TGF) interfere with your overall success. Learn to forgive yourself, and then hold yourself accountable to get back on track.

If you find that at the assigned calorie level you are losing more than two pounds per week after the first few weeks, you are too low on calories. Strive to lose from one half to one pound per week based on food intake alone. If you want to lose a bit faster, then increase your activity level. The calories cited for your gender, the weight you want to be, and age are an *estimate*. While pretty accurate, the table is not perfect in every case. The calories cited for the weight you want to achieve and maintain are making the assumption that you are lightly active on a daily basis. If this is not the case, you may need to increase or decrease the calorie level accordingly. The main thing is that we want to lose fat, not muscle; you can only ensure that if you are losing slowly enough.

If you choose to count calories or use the BUC™ Plan, you will need to be vigilant to ensure you are receiving proper nutrition. Take a look at how the choice plans break out servings of legumes, grains, fruits, and vegetables for the calorie level you have chosen. These are the number of portions you should still strive to get in each day for good nutrition. Yes, you may have some days of making less than stellar choices; we all do. However, if you strive for optimal nutrition 100 percent of the time and achieve it 95 percent of the time, then you are being *successful*! Remember, you do not have to be *perfect* to be successful.

Also, please note that it is fine for you to have more non-starchy vegetables at any time. The quantities per serving shown are simply a marker for you to know approximately how many servings of vegetables you are getting in a day. There is no restriction on any non-starchy vegetable. And adding these vegetables to what you had already planned on eating will make it much easier to stick to the weight loss plan.

As with any diet plan, you should discuss it with your physician before you begin. Since the plan meets the guidelines of the American Heart Association, he or she will likely support you to begin. If your physician tells you that you won't get enough protein, he or she is absolutely wrong. Even if you have diabetes, you should have no trouble using this diet to lose weight and become healthier. If you do have diabetes, it is best to spread your food choices throughout each day consistently so that you have roughly the same amount of carbohydrate at the same meal each day. For example, have the same amount of carbohydrate from breakfast today to breakfast tomorrow, from lunch today to lunch tomorrow, etc. Then let your blood sugars tell you how your method is working for you. We will discuss this more extensively in the diabetes chapter.

If you have any health issue for which you are under a doctor's care, you should definitely consult your physician before embarking on any new diet.

To begin, the table below indicates what your weight goal for your height should be in order to obtain a BMI of less than 25. Find your height, and record the weight goal. You can choose a higher or lower goal with your physician's input. Keep in mind that a BMI less than 18.5 is not a healthy goal.

	5'0"	5'1"	5'2"	5'3"	5'4"	5'5"	5'6"	5'7"	5'8"	5'9"	5'10"	5'11"	6'0"	6'1"	6'2"	6'3"	6'4"
Weight in pounds for BMI<25	127	131	136	140	145	149	153	158	163	167	173	178	183	188	193	198	204

Now that you have your weight goal, use the table below to identify the number of calories you need in order to maintain that weight. On the left hand side, choose your gender and weight goal. On the top, choose your age group. Where these match up is the daily calorie intake needed to maintain that weight for your age and gender. Round that number to the nearest 100 calories. For example, if the calorie number is 1,825, round to 1,800. If the number is 1,850 or 1,875, round up to 1,900. Again, it is perfectly fine to change the calorie level if you find you aren't losing weight over time. This is a process for you to really get to know your body.

Approximate Calories to Maintain Weight								
	Age in Years							
Women	18-25	26-34	35-39	40-45	46-50	51-55	56-62	over 62
100-110lbs	1650	1625	1550	1525	1500	1450	1425	1400
>110-120lbs	1725	1675	1625	1600	1550	1525	1500	1450
>120-130lbs	1800	1750	1700	1675	1625	1600	1550	1525
>130-140lbs	1850	1800	1750	1725	1675	1650	1625	1600
>140-150lbs	1925	1875	1825	1800	1750	1725	1700	1650
>150-160lbs	2000	1950	1900	1850	1825	1800	1750	1725
>160-170lbs	2050	2000	1950	1925	1900	1875	1825	1800
>170-180lbs	2125	2100	2025	2000	1975	1925	1900	1850
Men								
>110-120lbs	1750	1675	1600	1550	1500	1450	1400	1350
>120-130lbs	1975	1900	1825	1800	1725	1675	1625	1575
>130-140lbs	2075	2000	1925	1875	1825	1775	1725	1675
>140-150lbs	2175	2100	2050	2000	1950	1900	1850	1800
>150-160lbs	2300	2225	2150	2100	2050	2000	1950	1900
>160-170lbs	2400	2325	2250	2200	2150	2100	2050	2000
>170-180lbs	2500	2425	2375	2325	2275	2225	2175	2125
>180-190lbs	2625	2550	2475	2425	2375	2325	2275	2225
>190-200lbs	2725	2650	2575	2525	2475	2425	2375	2325
>200-210lbs	2825	2750	2675	2625	2575	2525	2475	2425

From here, choose which strategy you would like to use to start: calorie counting, the 95% Vegan Food Choices™ plan or the 95% Vegan BUC™ Plan. You can use any of them and even change strategies any time you wish; it will not impact your weight loss success.

If you are going to follow the 95% Vegan Food Choices™ Plan or the 95% Vegan BUC™ Plan, locate your calorie level at the top of the following table. On the left hand side of the table are each food choice in your diet plan: legumes, grains, vegetables, fruits, fats, desserts, and condiments. Under your calorie level, you will find the daily allowances for each food choice group. For example, if your calorie level is 1,800, you will get four legume choices, six grain choices, four (or more, as we discussed) vegetable choices, three fruit choices, one dessert, and two condiment portions each day. If you choose to use the BUC Plan, the last row on the bottom will tell you how many BUCs you have in a day. For example, if you are at 1,800 calories, you will get 26 BUCs each day.

Calorie Levels														
	1400	1500	1600	1700	1800	1900	2000	2100	2200	2300	2400	2500	2600	2700	2800
Legume	3	4	4	4	4	5	5	6	6	6	7	7	7	7	7
Grain	4	4	5	6	6	6	6	6	6	7	7	7	8	8	8
Vegetable	4	4	4	4	4	4	5	5	5	5	5	5	5	5	6
Fruit	3	3	3	3	3	3	3	3	4	4	4	4	4	5	5
Fat	3	3	3	3	3	3	4	4	4	4	4	4	4	5	5
Dessert	0.5	0.5	0.5	0.5	1	1	1	1	1	1	1	2	2	2	2
Condiment	2	2	2	2	2	2	2	2	3	3	3	3	3	3	3
Choice BUCs per Day	20	22	23	24	26	28	29	30	33	35	37	39	41	43	44

Here are some basic rules and tips for whatever method you choose:

1. *At least* for the first month, weigh or measure all of your food servings to ensure you are not underestimating how much you are eating. Most people cannot estimate portion sizes well without having measured them for a while.

If you do choose to stop weighing and measuring at any point, keep an eye on your weight to ensure you are not underestimating your portion sizes.

2. Anything that goes into your mouth counts, except for the non-starchy vegetables and unlimited food lists. You can eat as much as you like from these lists. Since we are not cutting your calories to a level of starvation, you must be accurate in tallying what you are eating, or it will become easy to stop losing weight.

3. Tip: As for weighing yourself, do whatever works for your psyche. If you find weighing yourself every day helps keep you on track, then that is what you should do. If you would rather just let how your clothes fit be your guide, go right ahead, but weigh yourself sporadically to ensure your progress is indeed on track. There is no right answer. Do be aware that it is normal to hit plateaus. If you know you have been losing weight consistently up to that point, then be patient as your body readjusts and starts to lose weight again. If you know you have slacked off and that is the reason for the plateau, then just get back to being a bit stricter with yourself. If you know you have been absolutely on track up until that point with respect to your eating habits, wait a week or two. If you don't start to lose after two weeks, you may need to go to the next lower calorie level or increase your activity level.

4. Do not eat too much simple carbohydrate in the morning. Keep your carb intake to 15–30 gm total for breakfast. Since our blood sugars are highest in the morning due to normal circadian rhythm, adding too much carb on top of this can cause you to feel drained and hungry throughout the day. A good option is to have a high fiber cereal (10–15 gm fiber per serving) with some soymilk. This will keep you from feeling as if you are starving by lunch.

5. As far as emotional support goes, again, do what is best for your psyche. Many people encourage getting support from family or friends. However, in my experience, sometimes family and friends can unintentionally or intentionally try to sabotage your success. If that is more the case for you, then don't even tell them what you are doing. You are getting so many calories in a day, far more than most plans allow, that you will still be eating normally in front of family and friends, just making healthier choices. They won't even know you are trying to lose weight unless you tell them. Only seek support from those you know will support you.

6. If you are a woman and you and your husband or boyfriend are going to embark on this weight loss journey together, don't compare your weight loss in pounds to his. Men have a much greater percentage of body weight in water than do women, which is why they lose weight faster. It can be pretty discouraging to women if they compare their success in pounds to a male counterpart.

7. Tip: Don't go to bed hungry. Save some calories for a bedtime snack so you aren't lying in bed thinking about how hungry you may feel. Even just one grain choice and a cup of antioxidant-rich tea can make a difference.

8. If at any time you do feel hungry, use that as a cue to pat yourself on the back for your success. The truth is that if you are losing weight, you will feel hungry from time to time. Just keep in mind that the calorie level you are at is the one you need to get used to in order to maintain the weight you are striving for. As you lose weight and get closer to that goal, you will feel less and less hungry because you are approaching the weight that your calorie level is intended to maintain.

9. Once you achieve your target weight, stay on the same calorie level. If you continue to lose weight from there and you wish to do so, then keep right on going. A BMI of less than 25 is usually more weight than what is considered your ideal body weight (IBW),* so if you want to lose more weight, that is fine. A BMI within the range of 18.5–25 is considered normal, so if you reach the upper limit and want to continue losing weight, then that is fine too! Just keep in mind that it is not healthy to have a BMI of less than 18.5. Since you now know how to figure out what weight you would need to be to have a certain BMI, make that your goal weight if you wish. On the other hand, if you feel good at the weight you achieve to have a BMI of less than 25, stay on the same number of calories. If you find you are continuing to lose more weight, you can go to the next higher calorie level or even more from there if necessary.

10. Also keep in mind that BMI does not reflect the size of your frame (bone size and density) or if you are extremely muscular. If you find that you feel better at a BMI greater than 25, then by all means, discuss this with your doctor to get his or her recommendation. Remember, if your waist circumference is greater than 31.5 inches for a woman or greater than 37 inches if you are a man, then BMI is likely going to be accurate for you to use as a guide.

Now we can begin to construct a daily meal plan for you. Even if you have decided you want to count calories, please follow along here to ensure you begin by following a healthy plan

---

* Ideal body weight (IBW) can be calculated for women by allowing 100 lb for the first 5 feet of height, plus 5 pounds for each additional inch. For men, allow 106 lb for the first 5 feet and 6 lb for each additional inch. Add 10 percent more for a large frame and subtract 10 percent for a small frame.

for your food intake. Let's go through this example using 1,800 calories as your daily allotment. Suppose you decided you wanted to use the 95% Vegan Food Choices™ plan. Here are the steps you would take.

Step 1

The first thing you need to do is to understand how many servings of each food choice list you are allotted each day. In the case of 1,800 calories, the chart tells you that your allowance for each day is:

> 4 legume choice servings
> 6 grain choice servings
> 4 vegetable choice servings (more if you desire)
> 3 fruit choice servings
> 3 fat choice servings
> 1 dessert choice serving (200 calories)
> 2 condiment choice servings

Step 2

Next, go to Appendix 6 to examine examples from each food choice list to get an idea of what foods are contained in each list and the portion sizes for each serving. You would consider how these food choices would best fit into your reality. For example, if supper is your largest meal, you need to allot the choices necessary to most closely mimic your typical supper, understanding that the amount of food you typically eat will be cut a bit to suit the weight loss scheme.

Step 3

Now you would write out how you see your food choices playing out on a daily basis. There is no right answer here; remember, you need to work out these food choices in a way that will work for *you*. You are the one who needs to make this plan work over the long haul. Also remember that this calorie level is what you will likely need to maintain the weight loss long-term. Certainly you can make whatever adjustments you feel you need in terms of when you will eat what food choices, as long as you remain within the assigned calorie level (unless you aren't losing weight or are losing it too fast). If you take insulin, it would be best to discuss the layout of your food choices with a dietitian who specializes in diabetes education. For those who do not have diabetes, do remember that it is best to avoid creating insulin spikes by having too much carbohydrate at one meal. In our example, you will see how easy it is to eat five small meals per day to keep your energy level high without causing an insulin surge.

For the 1,800 calorie example, if you place your food choices throughout the day as follows, you likely would not feel very hungry because you have spread your carb intake out throughout the entire day.*

> Breakfast: ½ grain, 1 legume, 1 fruit
> Lunch: 2 grain, 1 legume, 1 vegetable, 1 condiment, 1 fruit, 1 fat
> Afternoon snacks: 1 fruit, 1 grain, ½ legume, 1 fat
> Supper: 1–1 ½ legume, 2–2 ½ grains, 3 vegetables, 1 fat, 1 condiment
> Bedtime snack: 1 dessert

This represents a good start, but I know I can reallocate at any time. It is just good to start with a roadmap. Also, it is okay to borrow food choices from one meal to another, if my day's meals dictate it is necessary.

---

* Note: if you were using BUCs™, they would be allocated in this example as three for breakfast, six for lunch, one for afternoon snack, thirteen for supper, and three for a bedtime snack, for a total of twenty-six.

Step 4

Now it is time to put real food to the food choices. Below is an example day for our 1,800 calories day. It is a simple example, not necessarily the healthiest, but realistic as you are just forging your way toward veganism. As you get better at preparing vegan cuisine, the daily meal plans will become healthier, and with more delicious food options!

Breakfast

½ cup Fiber One™ cereal (½ grain)
½ cup lite vanilla soymilk for cereal, 1 cup as a coffee lightener (latte) (1 legume)
1 oz raisins on cereal (1 fruit)

Lunch

1 soy-based veggie burger (1 legume)
1 whole grain hamburger bun (1 grain)
1 tomato—half sliced for burger, half for side salad (1 vegetable)
Iceberg lettuce, cucumber, and tomato side salad
2 Tbsp Kraft® Fat Free Catalina dressing for side salad (1 fat)
3 Tbsp catsup for burger (1 condiment)
1 nectarine (1 fruit)

Afternoon Snacks

1 small apple (around 3:00 p.m.) (1 fruit)
3 cups popped popcorn with 2 Tbsp nutritional yeast flakes (around 5:30 p.m.) (1 grain, ½ legume)

Supper

Vegan Mexicali TVP "Ground Beef"* (1–½ legume, 1 fat)
2 medium flour tortillas (2.5 grain)

Vegetable mixture to wrap into tortilla: tomatoes, orange, and yellow bell peppers, broccoli, lettuce, fresh cilantro (equivalent to three vegetable choices)

6 Tbsp salsa (1 condiment)
*See Appendix 5 for recipe

Bedtime Snack

¾ cup So Delicious® Soy Chocolate Peanut Butter Ice Cream (1 dessert, 200 calories)

If you add up all of the food choice servings, you will see this pattern fits exactly what I had outlined in the beginning.

Now let's look at how we can calculate the 95% Vegan Food Choices™ from a recipe. If you aren't good with math, please don't let this section scare you. I simply want to provide as much helpful information as possible.

Suppose we wanted to make a delicious and nutritious vegan blueberry cobbler.

Delicious and Nutritious Vegan Blueberry Cobbler

Preheat oven to 400°F

Makes 12 servings

1 cup whole wheat flour
6 cups blueberries
1 cup all-purpose flour
½ cup raw sugar
2 tsp. baking powder
1 cup water
1 tsp. fine sea salt
2 Tbsp Earth Balance® butter substitute
¼ tsp. baking soda

1 Tbsp raw sugar
¼ cup chilled Earth Balance® butter substitute
1 cup minus 2 Tbsp lite vanilla soymilk
2 Tbsp white vinegar

1. Mix together the lite vanilla soymilk and white vinegar. An easy way to do this is to measure the 2 Tbsp. white vinegar and put that in a measuring cup, and then pour in the soymilk until it reaches the 1-cup line. Set aside and allow to curdle. This will become vegan buttermilk.

2. Mix together whole wheat and all-purpose flours, baking powder, baking soda, and salt in a large bowl.

3. Using a pastry blender, cut the ¼ cup Earth Balance® butter substitute into the flour mixture until it looks like pea-sized pieces.

4. Make a well in the center of the flour mixture. Pour in the vegan buttermilk, and stir with a spoon until the dough comes together in a ball.

5. Roll dough up in wax paper and store in refrigerator while preparing the filling.

6. Mix blueberries, ½ cup of raw sugar, and water together in a large bowl.

7. Melt 2 Tbsp. Earth Balance® butter substitute in a ten-inch cast iron skillet over medium heat. Pour the blueberry mixture into the skillet, and bring to a simmer. Decrease the heat to low. Cook while stirring until liquid is reduced and the mixture is thick, about 15 minutes.

8. Remove the dough from the refrigerator. Gently drop large spoonfuls of dough evenly into the blueberry mixture. Sprinkle 1 Tbsp. of raw sugar on top. Do not mix.

9. Bake the skillet in the preheated oven until browned in 15–20 minutes. Remove from oven and allow to cool until just warm before serving.

Per serving:
Calories: 187
Fat (gm): 5
Carbohydrate (gm): 35
Protein (gm): 3
Fiber (gm): 4

One serving of this recipe equals one dessert choice. It is close to 200 calories per serving. While it doesn't match up on the macronutrients, it is fine. There are so many different desserts with different macronutrient values, and many of them will not match up exactly with the macronutrients listed for one dessert. As long as your portion doesn't exceed 200 calories, it is fine. If you have a lower calorie amount for the day, you may only get ½ a serving of dessert per day. This equals 100 calories, and you may use them however you wish.

But considering that this particular dessert does have some nutritional value, we can use other food choices to account for the many ingredients in this recipe. For example, it has fruit and whole wheat. So if we consider a fruit choice in a serving of this recipe, we can begin to subtract from the total nutritional information as follows:

	Calories	Fat	Carbohydrate	Protein
Total recipe:	187	5	35	3
1 Fruit Choice	60	0	15	0
Remaining	127	5	20	3
1 Grain Choice	110	1.5	20	4
Remaining	17	3.5	0	0
½ Fat Choice	25	3	0	0
Remaining	-8	0.5	0	0

So for one serving of this recipe, we could count it as one fruit, one grain, and half of a fat. No, the math doesn't work exactly; it almost never does. But this method gives us the opportunity to figure out how we can include different recipes to keep our lives interesting. Dietitians have used this method for decades to help patients fit their favorite foods into their specific diet so that they can live their lives and still be successful. Now you know how too! For more practice examples, see the recipes in Appendix 5. Try to estimate the food choices yourself to see if your estimates match up to what we have estimated.

Now that you know the complicated stuff, let's talk about how you can simplify your plan for your daily life. There are so many tricks you can use. For example, if you are using the BUC™ system, you can simply tick off your BUCs™ throughout the day with a pen and pad. If you need more of a visual, you can use coins for your BUCs™. For example, a nickel might count ½ BUC™ and a dime represents a full BUC™. Move them from one pocket to another as you use them throughout the day. If you are using the food choices, you can use different color dot stickers to represent each choice group. If you have a smartphone or tablet, you can use that to enter daily calories, food choices, or BUCs™. Whatever works for you and keeps you enthusiastic is what you should use.

As for days you will eat animal products, simply substitute 1 oz cooked meat or cheese or 1 egg for each serving of legumes. The rest of the day will remain the same. Your fat intake on those days will certainly be higher, but it is for only one meal per week. We don't need to get any more technical than that.

You probably have many beloved recipes from your omnivore days. The good news is that you do not have to give many of them up in order to remain 95% vegan. Turn the recipe into a vegan recipe by using vegan substitutes. For example, one egg can be replaced with 1 Tbsp ground flaxseed plus 3 Tbsp water. Cow's milk can be replaced with soymilk. There are many other substitutes in the book *The Complete Guide to Vegan Food Substitutions* by Celine Steen and Joni Marie Newman (see Appendix 1). You can also search the Internet for various vegan substitutes to try.

YOUR TURN: 7 DAYS OF MEALS

This just might be your favorite homework assignment. It is the one that will finally get you on your way to achieving your healthy weight goals with a 95% vegan diet. Appendix 7 will serve as a guide for you to construct a week of your vegan weight loss plan's meals. Using Appendix 6 for portion sizes of various foods in each food choice list, researching for yourself the nutrient content of any foods you are interested in that aren't on the list and using recipes as you like, construct a seven-day meal plan for your first week of moving toward your weight goal. Then, from your meal plan, construct your first grocery list too!

This venture may feel like a struggle in the beginning. Remember the adage, "Anything worth having is worth working for." You are taking charge of your nutritional health, which requires some work. There is no magic bullet. I promise you though that if you keep track of your calculations (you may want to write them into your own cookbooks for future reference), it will become second nature to you. You won't have to do this hard work forever. However, it is important for your health goals to have a firm grasp on how to devise a *healthy* vegan diet. Remember, this is going to be the *last* time you will try to lose weight and make healthy eating a normal habit!

PREDIABETES AND TYPE 2 DIABETES MELLITUS

· ·

In this section, I write straight from the heart. As a Certified Diabetes Educator (CDE), I am extremely passionate for people with diabetes. They never get a day off from diabetes. They are frightened. They often don't know what to do to better control their blood sugar. There are friends and family with good intentions but who also pass along folklore and questionable information. It is all so confusing, and in that confusion stands a real live human being, who just wants it to go away. But the reality is that there is no known cure for type 2 diabetes. Your body cells have a defect that won't allow them to use the insulin you make properly. Sure, gastric bypass and other surgeries have proven useful in controlling blood sugar, sometimes to the point of people believing they have been cured. But the reality is that the defect is still there and would happily rear its ugly head again if challenged.

It pains me to walk past the dialysis unit at my hospital and see the suffering brought on by years of poor diabetes and blood pressure control. I ache when I see the patients in their early fifties admitted to the ICU (Intensive Care Unit) with their first heart attack brought on poor control and poor diet. And I grieve for those who come in to have a foot amputated, brought on by years of poor control. These consequences are so avoidable for the majority of these people. Yes, it is true that there are some people who had poor control but somehow escaped these consequences in the same way that there are smoking alcoholics who live to be one hundred. It is also true that there are people who had pretty good control who then have some of these consequences. But realize that people at either end of that spectrum are in the minority. Whether or not you suffer from the complications of diabetes is *largely* controlled by how well you met the goals of good control over time.

That is not to say you must be perfect every day. None of us can be, and you should not send yourself on a major guilt trip when you aren't. Think about the best baseball batters. Do they hit a home run every time they get up to the plate? Of course not. In fact, they strike out more than they hit home runs. However, they hit so many home runs that they became legendary. We will discuss your goals for hitting metaphorical home runs a bit later. Let's first discuss some of the facts.

Along with the alarming prevalence of overweight and obesity in the United States, we have equally alarming statistics for the prevalence of type 2 diabetes. In fact, if you look at the trends, you will see that diabetes is in fact, very closely linked to obesity (figure 1). Just look at the change in the prevalence of obesity from 2004 to 2009, and then compare that to the change in the prevalence of diabetes in that same time frame. Just look at what we as a nation have done to ourselves in just five years! It is no wonder why healthcare costs have skyrocketed, with such expensive diseases associated with obesity and our unhealthy Western diet.

Figure 1

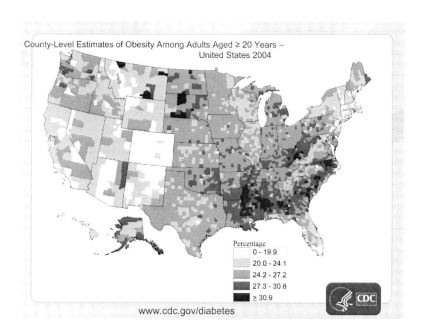

County-Level Estimates of Obesity Among Adults Aged ≥ 20 Years – United States 2004

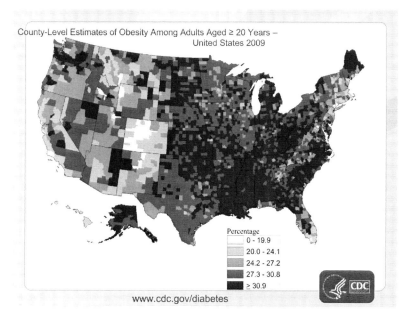

County-Level Estimates of Obesity Among Adults Aged ≥ 20 Years – United States 2009

(Figure 1 Continued)

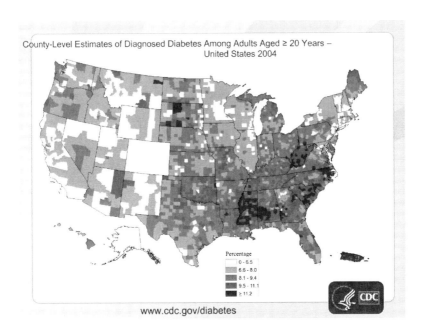

County-Level Estimates of Diagnosed Diabetes Among Adults Aged ≥ 20 Years – United States 2004

www.cdc.gov/diabetes

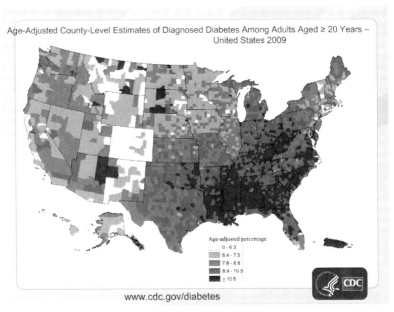

Age-Adjusted County-Level Estimates of Diagnosed Diabetes Among Adults Aged ≥ 20 Years – United States 2009

www.cdc.gov/diabetes

With the increasing prevalence of obesity in our youngsters, type 2 diabetes is showing up at a staggering pace in that population as well. The message is simple: *prevent obesity, prevent type 2 diabetes*. This is why I relentlessly preach the importance of creating a ripple effect for our future generations; it is far easier to prevent obesity than to lose weight. It is also easier to prevent type 2 diabetes than it is to live with it.

Type 2 diabetes accounts for 90 percent of all diabetes cases. While our genetics may predispose us to a stronger risk of developing diabetes, type 2 diabetes is in fact preventable. In a special issue of *The Lancet* (a world renowned medical journal) coinciding with the 70th Scientific Session of the American Diabetes Association, a very profound statement was made: "The fact that type 2 diabetes, a largely preventable disorder, has reached epidemic proportion is a public health humiliation."[1] The commentary also noted however that since type 2 diabetes is largely rooted in reversible social and lifestyle factors, a medical approach alone is unlikely to be the solution. It in fact suggested that by only focusing on the medical treatment of type 2 diabetes, we as healthcare providers are actually *disempowering* our patients. Healthcare providers should also pay attention to warning signs of disease in patients *before* the condition becomes full-blown. While many of them do address overweight and obesity in their patients, not all are necessarily diagnosing and letting patients know they have prediabetes. And many of those who are diagnosing prediabetes are not instilling the sense of urgency and the positive outlook of preventing type 2 diabetes as they should. However as we discussed before, physicians are already under pressure to economically sustain their practices *and* many patients do not seek out preventative health care.

So where does that leave us? In a nutshell, we usually only spend around fifteen minutes per year with our healthcare providers. This equates to not being with our healthcare providers around 99.997 percent of the time (really, do the math). This means that we are in charge of our own health destiny 99.997 percent of the time.

The prevention of diabetes lies within us as does the future health outcomes for those of us already diagnosed with diabetes.

Let's take a quick look at the most current CDC statistics (located at http://www.cdc.gov/diabetes/pubs/pdf/ndfs_2011.pdf):

- 25.8 million Americans have diabetes, but only 18.8 million have been diagnosed.

- 7 million Americans have diabetes but don't know it yet

- 79 million Americans 20 and older have prediabetes

How can you tell if you are one of the millions of Americans with prediabetes or diabetes? By simple blood sugar testing. Along with testing your blood sugar, your doctor may order an A1c test. The A1c reflects what your average blood glucose has been for the last two to three months. A1c levels can help confirm the diagnosis.

If your fasting blood sugar is 100–125mg/dl, that is called *Impaired Fasting Glucose* (IFG), which is prediabetes. If your two-hour postprandial (two hours after you eat) is from 140–199 mg/dl, this is called *Impaired Glucose Tolerance*, which is also prediabetes. You can go to almost any health fair to get this screening. Then it is up to you to see your physician in order to confirm the diagnosis.

Diabetes is often thought of as a disease of sugar; the blood sugar is too high. In fact, many people incorrectly believe that eating too much sugar causes diabetes. It does not. Unfortunately, diabetes is much more than that. It is a metabolic disorder that makes its victims much more prone to heart attacks, strokes, hypertension, chronic kidney disease, blindness, painful neuropathy (tingling and pain in the extremities), and amputations.

Approximately 80 percent of people with type 2 diabetes die of cardiovascular complications: heart attacks and strokes.

Since we are 99.997 percent in control of our destiny with diabetes and prediabetes, we have got to get a handle on how to manage the situation ourselves.

The presence of prediabetes (which has previously been called *borderline* diabetes, metabolic syndrome, and syndrome X) tells us that we must take control *immediately* in order to prevent the onset of type 2 diabetes. As we discussed earlier in this book, almost 60 percent of type 2 diabetes can be prevented through lifestyle changes (diet and exercise) *alone*. The medication known as metformin has been shown to prevent around 31 percent of type 2 diabetes.[2] This tells us that changes in diet and exercise habits are the *most* important influencers in the prevention of type 2 diabetes, almost twice as important as medication.

In fact, I would like you to think about prediabetes just as you would think of finding a malignant (cancerous) tumor. If you found a malignant tumor in your body, you would likely be sprinting to your physician's office to get treatment to prevent it from spreading throughout your body in order to increase your chances for survival. Since most people don't feel terrible with type 2 diabetes, they do not treat it with the same level of urgency when, in fact, they should. According to the American Diabetes Association's statistics, diabetes kills more people each year than breast cancer and AIDs combined; therefore, shouldn't we be treating it as if it were a terminal disease? Yes. And just because we don't always feel poorly with it, shouldn't we recognize that it is wreaking havoc within our blood vessels and organs? Yes. To do otherwise is called *denial*.

Whether you have been diagnosed with diabetes or prediabetes, the goals remain the same. In either instance, you are at a greater risk of death from cardiovascular disease. Fortunately, we do have set goals to strive for based on evidence-based medicine. This means that the cutoff limits for each goal are based on solid research that has informed us that any higher begins to create health issues or the *complications* of diabetes.

The following are the currently established goals for people with prediabetes or diabetes.[3] Meeting each of these gives you a metaphorical home run:

- Blood sugar: Before meals, the numbers are 70–130 mg/dl; two hours after meals: <180 mg/dl. These goals may be adjusted up or down by your physician depending on your individual health needs.

- A1c: < 7.0% (a goal of < 8.0% may be recommended for patients with a limited life expectancy and advanced complications of diabetes). Unless your A1c has been stable for a long period, you should have it checked every three months. It will not only confirm what your blood glucose meter is telling you; it will also let you know if you are having blood sugar problems during the day when you are not checking your blood glucose. It can also tell you if your blood glucose machine is not accurate. When it comes to A1c, the lower, the better.

- Blood pressure: No greater than 130 mmHg for systolic blood pressure and no greater than 80 mmHg for diastolic blood pressure, which is no greater than 130/80. If you have established kidney disease, your goals may be even lower, 125/75. Be aware that blood pressure control is every bit as important as blood sugar in preventing the complications of diabetes. As with blood sugar, you need to adopt a "whatever it takes" mindset for your blood pressure control. There is no shame in taking the medicines needed to control blood pressure. However, there *is* shame in having a heart attack or stroke because you didn't take the medicine you needed to control your blood pressure!

- Lipid (cholesterol) levels: LDL cholesterol is < 100 mg/dl (the goal may be set lower by your physician if you already have established heart disease). Triglyceride is < 150 mg/dl, HDL; cholesterol is >40 mg/dl (the higher the better). You may need medication to control one or more of these lipids.

- Exercise 150 minutes weekly (2–2 ½ hours or 30 minutes 5 times weekly). Ask your physician for recommendations as to what type of exercise would be best for you in your current state of health.

- Yearly musts include checking your kidney function, having a comprehensive foot exam (you should also check your own feet daily to ensure there are no wounds), having a dilated eye exam by an ophthalmologist, and having a flu shot (unless you have a contraindication to the flu shot, such as you are allergic to eggs).

- Depending on your risk level for heart disease, your doctor may suggest taking a baby aspirin, up to half of an adult aspirin (162 mg) to reduce the stickiness of your blood.

If you can meet these goals, you will vastly improve your chances for a long, healthy life. *Measure, measure, measure* these parameters to be absolutely satisfied you are meeting the goals. If you are trying your best but are unable to meet your blood glucose goals, it may be time for your physician to adjust your medicines. This doesn't mean you are a bad person. Type 2 diabetes changes over time; your medicines must progress with changes in your body. Even those with well-controlled weight sometimes require increased doses of their diabetes medications.

It always amazes me when people tell me their diabetes is controlled through diet and exercise, yet they do not routinely monitor their blood sugar and don't know what their A1c is. I have never been able to get to the root of how these people are defining good control; it is something mystical in their minds not based in reality. It is like saying that your home doesn't have termites without having a termite inspection. In short, they really have no clue as to whether they are under control or not. They will usually say something along the lines of "My doctor said my numbers were good." This is really not acceptable. Since we own 99.997 percent of the disease, we really need to know and understand our own numbers. Also, what if your doctor thinks an A1c of 9.0 percent is okay? Is that okay with you? The same holds true for people who say, "I only take one pill to control my diabetes." This tells me that they are defining how bad they think their diabetes is by the medicines they take. People who define their level of diabetes control by some mystical sense or by pill counting or whether or not they have to take insulin are frankly on the road to self-destruction. Their heads are in the sand. They are in denial.

But a word I would like to have with family and friends of people who have been diagnosed with diabetes or prediabetes is this: stop nagging. It is completely counterproductive and may even sabotage the patient's success *and* your relationship. Adults who have diabetes are just that: adults. We as adults are free to make our own choices when it comes to our health. Respect your friend/family member's rights and wishes. Let them know you care about the future of their health, that you are there for them and support their choices. Then just love them for who they are. In my career, I have seen so many patients who self-sabotage because they resent the nagging they receive. Allow them their time of denial. It is normal, and you would surely have it too given the same circumstances. Also, unless you have a clear scientific basis for any advice you want to give a family member, don't give it. A great deal of misinformation and old wives' tales exist about diabetes, and you can unintentionally add to your relative or friend's confusion and fear about controlling their diabetes.

If you have diabetes and have been nagged, feel free to show the perpetrator(s) this section.

Another word I would like to have, this time with people who already have signs or complications from poor blood sugar control is this: you aren't dead yet, and the recommendations provided by the American Diabetes Association can also slow the progression of these complications. It is not too late, so please keep trying!

Now for really good news. The ADA's nutritional recommendations are no different than what each of us (whether or not we have diabetes) should be doing for optimal health. You just have one more reason than those without diabetes to follow a healthy diet. The low fat, calorie-restricted diet I presented to you in the weight loss section is one of the strategies the ADA supports. The only thing that may be more important for you than for someone without diabetes is that it would behoove you to spread out your carbohydrate intake in a manner that is consistent from day to day. Not eating the same exact foods but roughly having the same number of grams of carbohydrate from breakfast to breakfast, from lunch to lunch, etc. can really help you get a handle on getting your postprandial blood sugars under control. For example, if I have one grain for breakfast every morning and check my blood sugar two hours after eating breakfast, my blood sugars should be fairly consistent at that same time every day if my medications and activity level were the same. By keeping your carb intake consistent, you can hit home run after home run. It will also help you see how other factors can impact your blood sugar. If you were to exercise one day and not the next, you will very likely see a difference in your blood sugars you would know were impacted by that exercise. If you forgot to take your diabetes medication (if you are on medication), you would see a difference you could attribute to your medicine. It is just easier to learn more about your body and your diabetes and how to control it when you can keep your carb intake consistent. Again, if you take insulin, I highly recommend you work with a diabetes dietitian to determine how best to space out your carbohydrate intake throughout the day.

If you need to lose weight and have not yet read the weight loss chapter and completed the Homework, please do so now. If you don't need to lose weight, please go to the weight loss chapter and find the number of calories needed to maintain your current weight. Then go through the rest of the weight loss chapter and complete the Homework, using your maintenance calories. Once you have completed your seven-day meal plan, come on back to this chapter for further instructions.

Assuming you have completed the Homework from the weight loss chapter, we will move on to the next steps toward better diabetes control moving forward.

Again, the only way to know if your diabetes is under good control is to *measure*. If you do not have a glucose meter, the first thing you will need to do is to get one. It is possible to obtain a meter free of charge by contacting the meter company. However, you should first find out from your health insurance company which meters' strips they will pay for. Many insurance companies only support one type of meter, and you cannot interchange strips from one meter to another. Once you find out what your insurance company will pay for in terms of strips, you can then work to get the meter free. Companies who make blood glucose meters don't make that much money from the meters; they make their money from the strips. Therefore, you may be able to contact the company and request a free meter. Simply search for the meter company online, and see their current offers for the meters themselves. Your pharmacy may also have deals on meters, so you may want to check there as well. Be sure you have a lancing device to obtain the drop of blood in the least painful way possible. Most lancing devices have different settings on them so that you can set the device to the shallowest depth possible for your fingertips while still allowing you to collect the drop of blood needed to check your blood sugar. Those with calloused fingertips will need to increase the depth to get the drop of blood. Be sure to obtain plenty of lancets and strips to check your blood sugar seven times per day for the first few weeks.

Homework: Your Diabetes Snapshot [Appendix 8]

The goal here is to discover any *patterns* in your blood glucose measurements for which adjustments may be needed. This is *not* a pass/fail test; it is simply *checking* to see where you are in terms of control.

For at least two weeks, check your blood glucose immediately before and two hours after breakfast, lunch, and dinner, as well as at bedtime, for a total of seven times per day. Record all readings as suggested in Appendix 8. In this way, you will see how each meal is impacting your blood sugar. You will also see if what you are eating is *consistently* pushing you out of control. While you may see a less than stellar reading on a day, if it doesn't happen on a consistent basis, we would not change anything about your diet or medications. Remember, you will be keeping your carbo-hydrate intake the same from breakfast-to-breakfast, lunch-to-lunch, etc. In this way, you can see if your decisions are optimal for your blood glucose control. If, after three days a certain meal's amount of carbohydrate has consistently caused a postprandial (two hours after you eat) glucose reading that is unacceptable (greater than 180 mg/dl), take some of the carbohydrate out of that meal and put it into another meal or add a snack with that carbohydrate. Placing exercise at the time of day you are having an issue may also help, if that is possible. Also, note what day of the week you are checking. Many people have different routines on their days off than on days they are working. Engaging in yard work or house cleaning when you are usually sedentary at work will usually yield lower blood sugars. The point is, you want to get to know your body and your diabetes to the point where you truly understand why you are having highs or lows.

On the subject of highs and lows, it is important to understand that you will likely only have lows if you are on a medication that can cause low blood sugars. Not all diabetes medicines can cause low blood sugars. However, as your blood sugar comes under better control, you may actually feel as if you are having a low blood sugar, even if you do not take medicine. It is important not to treat a feeling of being low unless it is *possible* you are low. Discuss your medications with your physician to understand if they can cause you to go too low. Whatever the case, it is always best, if possible, to check your blood sugar before eating anything to treat a low blood sugar. If you check your glucose and you are not low, it is best not to eat anything, or you will never get used to having normal blood sugars. The feeling of being low will pass the longer you stay within a normal range.

If over the two weeks, after making the changes you believe are necessary to get your blood sugar readings where they should be you have not been successful, I strongly encourage you to schedule an appointment with your physician to discuss whether changes or additions in your medications may help you reach the targets. Frequently, patients will have elevated fasting (before breakfast) glucose levels they cannot get under control. This does not have anything to do with their carb intake but rather with the fact that their liver is releasing too much glucose during the night. In this case, only medication or weight loss will get that reading to target. Remember, you need to take the "whatever it takes" approach to taking control of the situation and moving forward positively. You can do it!

After the weeks of checking your blood sugar seven times daily, if most of your readings are within the target limits, you can reduce the number of times you check your glucose daily. You may wish to check before and two hours after one meal daily, just to ensure you are remaining within the window of control. You must rotate which meal it is you are checking each day in order to ensure you are controlled all throughout the day. For example, on one day check before and two hours after breakfast; the next day, check before and two hours after lunch, and the next day, check before and two hours after dinner. If you were to check around the same meal each day, you would likely make the adjustments necessary to achieve control around that one meal, but then come out of control around other meals. The next thing you know, your A1c would be out of control, and you would have no clue why. If ever you were in that position, simply go back to the seven times per day exercise to identify the patterns contributing to your high A1c. It is so exciting to see your A1c go down and validate your hard work!

If your diabetes becomes more complicated to manage than what this chapter covers, work with your physician and a Certified Diabetes Educator to identify your needs to keep it under control. Please always remember that it does not matter what medication or how many medications it takes to keep your blood glucose under control, just that your blood glucose *is* under control.

CARDIOVASCULAR DISEASE

• •

Cardiovascular disease refers to all diseases of the heart and blood vessels. Hypercholesterolemia (high blood cholesterol), coronary plaque (blockages in the blood vessels to the heart), heart arrhythmias, heart failure, myocardial infarction (heart attack), and ischemic stroke (this type of stroke is due to a blockage of one or more blood vessels supplying the brain) are all encompassed in the term cardiovascular disease. We have discussed the benefits of moving to a plant-based diet to help prevent the onset of significant cardiovascular disease. In this section, we will discuss further the statistics in the American population and the nutritional guidelines from the American Heart Association— the foremost authority of evidence-based medicine for the heart.

Cardiovascular disease is the #1 cause of death in the United States. From the last published statistics of the American Heart Association (AHA), an average of 1 death every 37 seconds from cardiovascular disease occurs in America.[1] Of the 150,000 Americans who died in 2005 from cardiovascular disease, approximately 25,500 were less than sixty-five years of age. And in fact, the surgeon general has asserted that today's youth may be the first generation to not outlive their parents![2] Clearly, we have been heading in the wrong direction for the last couple of generations (about fifty years). If we begin to turn the tide *now*, it will likely still take two full generations to reverse the trend, but a huge impact can be made in our own lifetime. If those of us who grew up in the sixties or earlier don't share how we grew up with healthy portion sizes and balanced meals with our children and grandchildren, creating that ripple effect will be even more difficult, since the two generations following that era were not necessarily raised with this knowledge and self-control.

The American Heart Association's nutritional guidelines' emphasis is on dietary management to achieve and maintain a healthy weight and optimal cholesterol, glucose, and blood pressure levels.[3] The importance of avoiding tobacco products and engaging in regular physical activity are also emphasized. The practical implementation tips emphasize reducing fat by choosing lean meats and dairy products, an issue we as vegans generally do not have to concern ourselves with. However, it is possible to have an unhealthy vegan diet by eating too many nuts and adding too much fat to our food. While the monounsaturated fat from nuts is certainly better than the saturated fat from meat and dairy products, if you have elevated cholesterol levels, no fat is a good fat, except for the minimal amount of the essential fatty acids we require as discussed in the macronutrient section.

For those who have hypertension (high blood pressure), the DASH diet (**D**ietary **A**pproaches to **S**top **H**ypertension) is recommended by the AHA. If you look at the dietary recommendations of the DASH diet (available at http://www.nhlbi.nih.gov/health/public/heart/hbp/dash/new_dash.pdf), you will see that it emphasizes low sodium intake, 2,300 mg or less. This is extremely important since sodium increases water retention, which then increases how hard the heart has to work. If you can get lower than 2,300 mg, that would be even better. For the DASH diet's recommendations for lean meat and fat-free or low-fat dairy, you could as a vegan substitute legumes to ensure adequate protein intake. Ensuring you burn as many calories as you eat will maintain your current weight, and eating less than you burn will cause you to lose weight. The weight loss section of this book absolutely meets the DASH diet's requirements, provided you do not add salt.

The truth is that a healthy vegan diet very easily meets all of the AHA nutritional guidelines, provided you reduce your sodium intake to 2,300 mg or less and do not add fat excessively. In fact, a vegan diet can completely rid your diet of the saturated fat you would get from the DASH diet's meat allowance.

The most important thing for you to remember is that your #1 goal is to achieve the targets set by the AHA for cholesterol levels and blood pressure goals. If your blood pressure is at or above 120/80 (120 mmHg systolic blood pressure and 80mmHg diastolic blood pressure), you need to take action. Weight loss and sodium control can certainly help you lower blood pressure, but if you cannot meet the goal of *less than* 120/80 *consistently*, you will very likely need to take medication to achieve the targets. Please do not resist taking medication if you need it to achieve target goals. There is no shame in taking medication to achieve the targets, but there *is* shame in ignoring the issue and having a heart attack or stroke because you refused to take medication.

The same goes for cholesterol goals, which vary based on your risk level for having a cardiac event.

Risk Category	LDL Goal	Initiate Therapeutic Lifestyle Changes	Consider Drug Therapy
High Risk (10-year risk >20%)	<100mg/dl	≥100mg/dl	≥100mg/dl
Moderately High Risk (10-year risk10%-20%)	<130mg/dl	≥130mg/dl	≥130mg/dl
Moderate Risk (10-year risk<10%)	<130mg/dl	≥130mg/dl	≥160mg/dl
Lower Risk(10-year risk <10%, and 0-1 risk factors)	<160mg/dl	≥160mg/dl	≥190mg/dl

> Adapted from The National Cholesterol Education Program Report: Implications of Recent Clinical Trials for the National Cholesterol Education Program Adult Treatment Panel III Guidelines.
> Endorsed by the National Heart, Lung, and Blood Pressure Institute, American College of Cardiology Foundation, and American Heart Association. Circulation, 2004; Vol. 110, pp. 227-239.

The medications used to control cholesterol and triglycerides are very safe and have been on the market for decades. Again, while losing weight and increasing your exercise level can help correct cholesterol issues, they may not be enough to get you to the targets. If this is the case, be sure to work with your physician to get to the goals. It is not good enough to get it down; you must meet the targets that were set based on scientific evidence to ensure optimal health outcomes.

As with diabetes, people with high blood pressure and cholesterol issues do not feel badly until the heart attack or stroke hits. This is why heart disease is called the *silent killer*. You should begin to have your fasting lipid profile drawn by age twenty and a minimum of every five years thereafter. If you have a strong family history for heart disease, your physician may recommend you have it checked more often. Pay close attention to your numbers, and treat them as if they were a cancer that needs to be cut out; maintain a sense of urgency to eradicate the problem. That is the best you can do. I lost both of my parents unexpectedly as a result of cardiovascular disease. They ignored the warning signs and refused to take medicine for issues like mild hypertension and abnormal cholesterol levels. They never felt badly because of it but then left us tragically and suddenly due to their unfortunate decisions. While it is true that as adults we can choose our own health destiny, we need to do so with our eyes wide open to the risks of ignoring warning signals.

CHRONIC KIDNEY DISEASE

• •

Chronic kidney disease (CKD) is a progressive loss of kidney function. In the majority of cases (67 percent), it is caused by years of poor control of diabetes and/or hypertension.[1] Other causes include tumors, exposure to toxic chemicals, immunological diseases, congenital malformations, repeated urinary tract infections, and obstructions. CKD is irreversible, but there are steps one can take to prevent it from progressing.

CKD is defined in stages, based on the GFR (Glomerular Filtration Rate). In the "Laboratory Assessments for Nutritional Health Status" section, we discussed how to calculate your GFR. The stages of CKD are as follows[2]:

Stage	Description	GFR ml/min
1	Kidney damage with normal or increased GFR	≥90
2	Kidney damage with slightly decreased GFR	60-89
3	Moderately decreased GFR	30-59
4	Severely decreased GFR	15-29
5	Kidney failure/dialysis	<15

The main goal of treatment for all nondialysis stages is to prevent progression toward needing dialysis or a kidney transplant while maintaining an optimal nutritional status. As patients progress through the CKD stages, their kidneys lose the ability to maintain electrolyte and fluid balance, as well as acid:base balance. Large shifts in electrolytes, particularly potassium, can be life threatening. Frequent lab testing guides the nutritional and medication recommendations. Medications to correct anemia, bind phosphorous, and maintain micronutrient status are all very common in patients with kidney disease.

For all of the nondialysis stages, restriction of protein down to 0.6 gm/kg is important so as not to further tax the kidneys. Fluid intake should equal the amount of output of urine plus no more than one liter (slightly more than one quart). Restriction of potassium to 2–3 gm (2,000–3,000 mg), sodium to 2 gm (2,000 mg), calcium to no more than 2,000 mg elemental calcium, and phosphorous to 800–1,000 mg is also recommended.[3] Since meat and dairy are sources of huge quantities of protein, potassium, and phosphorous, following a 95% vegan diet may help with compliance to the recommended limits of these nutrients, provided you also avoid those fruits and vegetables that are high in potassium.

Fruits and vegetables to avoid are tomatoes, bananas, orange juice, prunes and other dried fruits, potatoes (both white and sweet), and melons (cantaloupe and honeydew).

Grains to avoid are whole grains, brown rice, high-fiber muffins, and salted crackers.

Legumes to avoid are dried beans and peas (use canned instead, as the canning process leaches out potassium), nuts, and seeds. Read labels to ensure a low sodium intake. Other foods to avoid include chocolate, beer, and cola sodas.

It is important to read food labels to ensure you maintain the recommended limits listed above. But the good news is that since you are already cutting out meat and dairy, staying within the limits will be much easier. I strongly recommend you work closely with your physician to keep a close watch on your kidney function, electrolytes, and nutritional status.

If you take any type of medication and discover your GFR to be less than 60 ml/min, it is important to consult with your physician or pharmacist to determine if you should reduce the dose of any of your medications or stop taking them altogether. This includes over-the-counter medications as well. For example, people with significant kidney disease should avoid taking ibuprofen though it is one of the most frequently used over-the-counter medications used. Do not stop taking any of your scheduled medications without first discussing it with your physician.

CELIAC DISEASE

Celiac disease, also called sprue, is both an immune and autoimmune disease involving the small intestine. A complex interaction between gluten from wheat, rye, barley, and the individual's genetic makeup and other immunological factors create inflammation in the small intestine. This inflammation can lead to malabsorption of macro- and micronutrients.[1] This can lead to malnutrition, characterized by weight loss, low serum albumin, anemia, and bone disease.[2] Celiac disease can present with intestinal symptoms and sometimes with an itchy skin rash. It is diagnosed through specific antibody testing and sometimes confirmed with an intestinal biopsy.

Treatment of celiac disease requires a strict, lifelong, gluten-free diet. In addition, any nutritional deficiencies or bone disorders need to be identified and treated. I strongly recommend that those with celiac disease consider joining a celiac support group in order to more quickly learn how to live and adhere to a gluten-free diet. Also, www.celiac.com has numerous gluten-free recipes that may be helpful.

More and more gluten-free food products are rapidly entering the marketplace. Many of these items are also vegan.

Whether or not you have celiac disease should not be a factor in deciding to strive for a 95% vegan diet. Beans, peas, and pea flours are all gluten-free, as are vegetables and fruits.[3] Plain tofu is also gluten-free. Grains and cereals prepared from corn, potato, rice, or soy flour are gluten-free. Millet, kasha (buckwheat groats), quinoa (pronounced "Ken-Wah"), and tapioca are gluten-free. Oat products not contaminated with gluten-containing products are gluten-free. You will need to read food labels to ensure that traditionally gluten-free foods have not had a gluten-containing product added. You will also have to avoid the vegan meat recipes that call for vital wheat gluten, but there are so many other options to please the palate on a vegan diet; don't let that dissuade you from following the healthiest gluten-free diet on the planet!

DIVERTICULOSIS

Small pouches of weakened tissue in the large intestine that bulge outward characterize diverticulosis. The small pouches are called diverticula. Having diverticula becomes more common as we get older; about 10 percent of people over forty years of age have it, and almost half of all people over the age of sixty have it.[1] Symptoms of diverticulosis are usually fairly mild, mainly bloating and constipation.

Diverticulitis occurs when there is an acute inflammation of the diverticula; the pouches become inflamed. In other words, the diverticula that were already there have become inflamed for some reason. It can lead to infections, perforations (tears), and bowel obstruction. The symptoms of diverticulitis are far more pronounced and may even require a hospital stay for IV antibiotics, total parenteral nutrition, and management of pain.

The treatment of *diverticulosis* (the *non*inflamed state) is a high fiber diet. Fiber in the diet helps to move food through the intestinal tract more quickly, thus preventing deposition and retention of food particles in the small pouches, which can cause an acute flare-up of diverticulitis. Physicians often also recommend taking a fiber laxative two to three times per day, with at least 8 oz of water. It is very important to keep fluid intake high with a high fiber diet to facilitate its passage through the GI tract. There are many vegan fiber laxatives available on the market.

The treatment of diverticulitis (the inflamed state) is quite different. If severe and the patient is hospitalized, he or she may not be able to take anything by mouth at all. This then requires nutritional intervention through the intravenous route. As the inflammation subsides, the patient is then moved to clear liquids (water, broths, and popsicles) then to a bland diet. Four to six weeks after the diverticulitis subsides, the patient is prescribed a high fiber diet again in an attempt to avoid future flare-ups. At that point, a minimum of 25 grams of fiber and a minimum of 2 quarts of water should be consumed daily (unless there are other confounding medical ailments that need to be considered).[2]

Given the treatment for diverticulosis is a high fiber diet, it makes good sense to move forward with your plans for becoming 95% vegan, being particularly mindful of achieving the fiber and water intake recommendations. During diverticulitis flare-ups, stay away from all products with significant fiber content. Instead, stick with clear liquids such as vegan broths and fruit juice popsicles without pulp. When you are up to it, you can progress to full liquids such as nondairy milks, vegan ice creams, and the like. From there when you are up to it, you can add bland, soft foods such as soft white bread, white rice, and tapioca. Anything that doesn't worsen the flare-up and has little or no fiber is fine. The goal is to keep the flare-up from becoming so serious as to require a hospital stay, if possible. Of course you should consult your physician if you have any questions or the symptoms are severe.

PART 5:
Become Your Own Scientist

Now we come to the part that the dietary supplement doesn't want you to know about. It is a multibillion-dollar industry with a huge lobbyist presence in Washington, D.C., designed to keep the government from regulating it as it does the pharmaceutical industry. As you will see, the dietary supplements you find at health food stores do not have to pass the rigorous scientific scrutiny that drugs do in order to make it to the market and stay there. These supplements are a special category of foods and have flexible and lenient rules for regulation. The term *supplement* is broadly defined to include herbs, amino acids, vitamins, enzymes, organ tissues, metabolites, extracts, or concentrates—anything that supplements the diet.

As you may already know, we are finding that even drugs that passed the initial rigorous scrutiny required to get to the market are sometimes found to have complications that were not seen in the clinical drug trials. For example, Vioxx®, an anti-inflammatory drug used in arthritis, was pulled from the market following thousands of heart attacks and sudden deaths. Rezulin®, a drug for type 2 diabetes, was pulled from the market following a number of cases of liver failure. There are many other examples of drugs that made it to market, only to find out they weren't safe. Clinical drug studies are very short in comparison to how long patients with chronic diseases will use them during their lifetime. The point is, even highly regulated, well-studied medications slip through the cracks of safety, in spite of the scientific evidence required to get them to market. How on earth would you know if a dietary supplement or herbal remedy is safe to begin with, let alone its long-term safety, if it isn't even studied rigorously to make it to the market in the first place? The answer is, you really won't know, unless it becomes sensational news.

The mistakes that become the misfortune of people who regularly use these leniently regulated substances is that they assume the following:

1. Because they are over-the-counter products, they must be safe.

2. "Natural" and herbal products must be safe and good for them.

3. The government regulates these products like they do medicines.

4. The people who are selling these products have formal education from accredited institutions. Since they can spout off information (whether scientifically credible or not) they are to be believed.

5. The herbal remedies and supplements they buy are of a guaranteed potency, and do not contain any harmful contaminants. (There have been several findings that prove this to be untrue.)

In fact, many toxic side effects from the herbs themselves have been reported, as have adverse events from contaminants and herb-prescription drug interactions.[1] Herbal and other dietary supplements can be just as dangerous as FDA approved medications. On the flip side, many FDA approved drugs originally come from plants and herbs. Some examples include quinine, a malaria drug being extracted from the bark of the cinchona tree; digoxin, a heart medication being extracted from foxglove (digitalis purpurea); and vincristine, a drug used to treat cancer, comes from the Madagascar periwinkle.

Plants and herbs used for drugs have just been reduced to a concentrated tablet or capsule form to make pharmaceutical dosage strengths. However, keep in mind the following:

1. These plant-based drugs have been rigorously tested for efficacy and safety before entering the market.

2. Pharmaceuticals rarely contain any drug substance other than legally approved products. Many dietary supplements have been found to contain unapproved drug substances.

3. The herb in question has been concentrated into pharmaceutical strengths that have demonstrated efficacy. Although an herbal product may contain the labeled product, how do you know it is in a strength that will have a positive impact on your health?

You may be surprised to know that only in 2012 has the FDA moved toward prioritizing the monitoring of drugs *after* they get to the market in the same manner as they monitor safety in premarket drugs (see April 21, 2012 news release at http://www.fda.gov/NewsEvents/Newsroom/PressAnnouncements/ucm301165.htm).

If we are so far behind in this important step for FDA approved drugs, how far behind are we for the dietary supplement industry?

As you will see in the next chapter, the FDA has the burden of proof to demonstrate that an herbal remedy is *not* safe in order to remove it from the market, as opposed to drug manufacturers having to prove a drug is safe and effective *before* it can be marketed in the United States. In other words, the general public is the supplement industry's guinea pigs. Only when there have been enough reports to prove the product is unsafe can the FDA make a move. One particularly grisly example of the potential toxicity of an herbal supplement occurred in Belgium with a Chinese herbal product for weight loss. The product contained an herb called *Aristolochia fangchi*. Forty-three patients developed end-stage kidney disease, and thirty-nine had their kidneys removed prophylactically (to prevent other potential dangers). Eighteen of the patients were found to have a type of cancer called urothelial carcinoma.[2]

A more recent example in the United States involved another Chinese herb called ma huang, also used for weight loss. Ma huang contains ephedra, which is chemically similar to amphetamine (also known as "speed" on the street). It raises heart rate and blood pressure, sometimes dangerously so, resulting in heart attacks, stroke, and sudden death. Although it became popular in the United States in the 1990s, it could not be removed from the market until 2004. First, it was discovered that there are forty times the number of calls to poison control centers concerning ephedra compared to other herbal products.[3] Then there was a meta-analysis of studies comparing ephedra to placebo for weight loss and performance enhancement.[4] That systematic review revealed that people who took ephedra were 2.2 to 3.6 times as likely to have psychiatric and gastrointestinal symptoms (nausea and vomiting), as well as heart palpitations. The total combined evidence against the safety of ephedra finally enabled the FDA to remove it from the market in 2004.

What is particularly bothersome is that supplement manufacturers quickly worked to replace the lost income from ephedra by then marketing products with the herb *Citrus aurantium* and caffeine. The herb, also known as bitter orange, contains synephrine, which has a chemical structure similar to ephedrine, and can cause the same cardiac effects. Not unexpectedly, this herb is touted as an ancient Chinese herb used for thousands of years in traditional Chinese medicine. However, this herb actually made it to the *Consumer Reports* "Dirty Dozen Supplements" and for good reason. It has caused cardiac arrhythimias, heart attacks, stroke, and death.

There is one simple question to ask yourself when it comes to claims of weight loss supplements: "If the product is that good, why isn't it being marketed as a drug?" Pharmaceutical companies have been falling all over themselves trying to get weight loss drugs to the market for years and years, knowing the potential market and billions of dollars a proven product would make. However, in well-designed clinical trials, the drugs are found to either not work or cause intolerable side effects. They cannot pass the tests necessary to gain FDA approval. Knowing that supplements have no such research going into them, what do you think the likelihood of one of them passing the FDA tests would be?

With all that said, let me be very clear that it is not that I don't believe there are any good dietary supplements out there that may work well for you. I am agnostic when it comes to dietary supplements; just show me through good science that they are safe and effective for whatever they are being touted for.

Have you ever heard the term *placebo effect*? It is a phenomenon that is routinely observed in well-conducted clinical trials whereby patients with the studied ailment who are receiving the placebo (which is the inactive product often called the sugar pill, injection, or solution) actually get better. Placebos are designed to look exactly like the active drug and are used in double-blind clinical studies in order to credibly study the effects of the active drug being studied. Although patients sign an informed consent document, which informs them of their chances of getting placebo, they may believe that the placebo is the real drug. In addition, some conditions, even cancers, can get better for a short period, which also adds to the placebo effect. In fact, placebo works to improve a patient's ailment about 33 percent of the time! It speaks loudly of the mind-body connection. If one believes a remedy will work it is likely that they will feel the effects they believe the remedy will have on them. And since the dietary supplement industry isn't held to the same controlled clinical trial standards with reproducible results, it is likely that many people are actually spending their money to achieve the placebo effect. This is why it is extremely important that you understand the science that went into (or didn't) the claims being made about a given product. We are going to discuss what makes good science and look at some of the products on the market in order to help you see the difference. In the end, it is your choice about what you choose buy and put inside your body, but you should do so as a well-informed consumer.

WHAT IS GOOD SCIENCE?

. . . .

There are scores of books on the subject of what makes good science. The subject is highly technical, but the bottom line is simple:
*if we understand how to spot questionable science, we can protect our
health and not waste money on unproven products.* It is very important to keep in mind that whenever you hear the term "clinical
studies *prove*," you should immediately be suspicious. By nature,
that claim is almost always an overstatement. A more appropriate claim would be something along the lines of "Clinical studies support the efficacy and safety of (*insert name)* for treating
ailment XYZ." No product is a panacea. Every drug and every
supplement should be specific in what they are indicated to treat
or support. However, even if the statement was more tempered,
because dietary supplements are not held to rigorous scientific
standards of reputable research to begin with, you should still
temper your enthusiasm until you actually know how the studies
were conducted. Multiple, scientifically valid, extremely expensive (in the tens of millions of dollars) studies on large study
populations would have to all provide the same results in order to
make the statement "clinical studies prove" with credibility. Since
the herbal/dietary supplement industry is not required to make
such an investment, they don't. The first thing you should *always*
ask a salesperson that makes that sort of claim is, "Where were
the clinical studies published?" If they can't tell you, your level of
suspicion should rise considerably because you just caught that
person spouting off nonsense that they can't back up with solid

information about the source of information. That is a *salesperson*, not a credible healthcare professional. If the person does seem to have a legitimate response, ask them to kindly provide you the citations (references) so that you can read the studies yourself. If the salesperson has the information available to back up their statement, they will generally share it gladly. If they don't know or have the information, you can expect them to become defensive or make excuses.

Not too long ago, a colleague of mine was touting a new diet supplement that several physicians in the area were starting to sell in their offices. My colleague provided me the references to the "clinical studies" that were completed on the product. And even though a couple of the references were published in well-known, peer-reviewed journals, the studies themselves were negative; they actually showed the product didn't work. But because the company selling the product could spout off these references, they did so, apparently not expecting anyone to check the studies. Sadly, several physicians in the area were then selling the garbage to their own patients! The point is, no one is immune from being sold something if the salesperson is convincing enough, not even physicians or other healthcare providers.

In order to discuss the basic principles of what good clinical research looks like, we will need to more closely examine the gold standards of good science. The following are terms to help you decide whether to believe the studies behind a product are based in solid scientific principles.

"Prospective" means the study was designed in advance as opposed to haphazardly observing effects after they have occurred. If a study is prospective, it should state up front one or more hypotheses that were going to be studied, in advance of conducting the study. A hypothesis is an educated guess about how the study will turn out. An example would be "Drug A will not be inferior to drug B in improving knee pain experienced following knee replacement surgery." Noninferiority simply means that the drug will perform at least as well as the comparator. Then the statistics explaining how the pain will be measured, collected, analyzed, interpreted (how the claim of noninferiority will be established), and presented are defined and stated in advance.

"Statistically significant" refers to whether an observed difference occurred due to chance alone or if the difference was truly caused by a difference in effect of the studied product. In valid scientific studies, the measure of statistical significance is decided in advance. For example, let's say we are going to test the hypothesis that smoking more than one pack of cigarettes per day for ten or more years is associated with a statistically significant increase in the incidence of lung cancer in the U.S. population. We would formulate a traditional hypothesis, called the "null hypothesis," which would state that we expect *no* difference (null) among smokers and nonsmokers with respect to the incidence of lung cancer in two similarly matched groups of people. (I know this doesn't seem to make any sense, but this is how it is done.) Since we can't study all of the people in the United States, we would take a representative sample of the population who has smoked more than one pack of cigarettes per day, as well as a representative sample of the population who have never smoked. We would then decide what the cutoff would be in terms of how much more lung cancer we would have to see in the smoking group population in order to reject the null hypothesis and accept that there is a difference in the incidence of lung cancer in people who smoke more than one pack per day over ten or more years. The *p-value* tells us the probability of observed differences being due to chance alone. It tells us whether the results we are seeing are within the expected *confidence interval* or not. The confidence interval is a predefined range of expected observations if a given study was repeated many times. In science, we generally assume that if the p-value is greater than 5 percent ($p > 0.05$), there is no significant difference between the studied groups and the observed difference is due to chance alone. In general, only if the p-value is less than or equal to 5 percent ($p \leq 0.05$) would we state there is a statistically significant difference. If $p \leq 0.05$, we would reject the null hypothesis that there is no difference between the smokers and nonsmokers and make the assumption that the observed difference was not due to chance but due to the biological effects of smoking. However, an important thing to note is that the smaller the sample (the number of people studied), the more likely there will be greater individual variability. This means that there would need to be much greater differences between the smokers and nonsmokers with respect to the incidence of lung cancer in order to validly claim the difference was not due to chance alone. This is why medically credible organizations require large studies before they will endorse a product or a concept—it is just too easy for smaller studies to appear that the product was significantly different.

"Clinically significant/relevant" is an important concept to understand too, in that although there may have been a mathematically statistically significant difference between two groups, the results may not necessarily be *clinically significant*, meaning that the difference observed is not strong enough to truly impact a patient's ultimate health outcome. For example, suppose a weight loss product claims a significant difference in its ability to help morbidly obese people lose weight. In reading the study, you see that a difference of ten pounds was what the investigator(s) decided was statistically significantly different. In reading further, you note that while the group taking the supplement lost, on average, ten pounds more than the comparator group, they still ended the study being morbidly obese. In other words, losing ten pounds more would not place them in a lower-risk category. We would then say that although the amount of weight lost was *statistically* significantly different, we would also conclude that the difference was not *clinically relevant*; the study group remained in the morbidly obese group, not significantly changing their risks for chronic diseases.

"Double-blind" means neither the patient nor the investigator know if the patient is getting active study drug, placebo, or an active comparator. (Active comparators are typically used in studies in which it would be unethical to treat patients with a placebo. For example, in cancer studies, we would give the control group whatever the standard of care is for a particular type of cancer and study another drug to see if it is better than the current standard of care.) The purpose of a study being double-blinded is so that bias is not introduced. For example, suppose a study is single-blinded, meaning that only the patient is unaware of what he or she is taking (active drug or placebo or comparator drug). The investigator (usually a physician) knows what the patient is taking but does not tell the patient during the course of the study. The investigator may have an opinion or have certain expectations about how the drug being studied or its comparator should affect the patient, so he or she may unintentionally bias the patient. For example, suppose the investigator is experienced in the area of diabetes. The investigator has used the comparator drug extensively in his practice and has often observed that patients seem to have excessive nausea from this comparator. By knowing this, the investigator may unwittingly probe the study patients more deeply for excessive nausea on the comparator versus the study drug. This in turn may signal to patients that they should feel nausea, and lo and behold, they actually do. It may well be that the study drug has an equal likelihood of causing excessive nausea, but the patients taking that drug do not report it as frequently because they aren't asked about it in the same way as the other group. The investigator has introduced a *bias* to the study results. This phenomenon occurs even more frequently in *open-label* studies because both the investigator and the patient know what the patient is receiving.

"Randomized" means that the study subjects were not cherry-picked to take the drug. Cherry picking is when patients are consciously chosen to take the drug, usually because the investigator believes the patients chosen are most likely to respond to the studied drug. You will see this done frequently in clinical studies conducted on dietary supplements. Randomization is like picking names out of a hat. Whether or not a patient is assigned to the drug, placebo, or an active comparator (usually a drug that works similarly to the drug being studied) is completely by chance alone. Cherry picking biases results because people will naturally choose the treatment they expect to be effective in the given patient population.

Having adequate numbers of study patients is critical for a scientifically credible study. A clue to determine whether a study had enough patients in each group to truly detect a scientific difference is how the study is *powered*. Powering is a measure of how great the ability of the study is to demonstrate statistical significance. In order to adequately power a study, an appropriate number of patients must be studied. Determining the total number of patients needed to adequately power a study is accomplished through precise mathematical calculations. Somewhere in the text of the study, it should state how well it was powered. A minimum acceptable powering is 80 percent. If a study doesn't state powering at all, be very suspicious. There are many studies out there that claim there was a statistically significant benefit for a product but the study really wasn't appropriately powered; there weren't enough subjects studied to make that claim with scientific credibility. Another clue here would be to look at the actual numbers of patients included. While you may not have the ability as a statistician does to determine if the study was adequately powered, if there are less than one hundred patients studied before the product was brought to market, it was likely not powered highly enough to provide scientifically valid results. My observation with most supplements is that they often have fewer than fifty patients in a single study, not exactly good science in general. Furthermore, be aware that from a strictly mathematical point of view, it becomes more difficult to demonstrate cause and effect with more patients than with fewer patients if there truly is no cause and effect there. Think about it. If you only have twenty patients in a study, ten in each group, and two patients in one group experiences a positive effect that no one in the other group experiences, the investigator can state that drug A is 20 percent more beneficial than drug B. While this may be true, only two patients had the experience; how would you know if it happened just by chance? Could those results be replicated in a larger population? With dietary supplements, since the companies do not have to invest in large clinical trials, they don't; you will likely never know if the results from those small studies could be replicated. On the other hand, if you have one hundred patients on each drug, you would have to see the effect in twenty patients for it to be meaningful, which is more difficult to accomplish.

"Controlled" is another important term to be familiar with. All good science has "controls" in place to ensure that other factors (also called variables) do not influence the results observed. A good example here is that both the study group and the placebo (or active comparator) group resemble each other. They are of similar age. They all have the condition studied; other clinical parameters such as baseline BMI (for diet supplements) are comparable. Also, there should be specific exclusions for factors that can influence the results. For example, in a weight loss study, any patients who may have uncorrected thyroid disease would be excluded from being in either group because the condition can influence the study results.

This is also a good place to revisit the concept of not being able to prove an effect by a product if too many variables are changing at the same time. For example, many well-known weight loss products provide a diet in their labeling for while a person is using the product. If you look closely, you can easily see that the recommended diets tend to be very low in calories. In other words, if you just followed the enclosed diet but never took the product, you would still lose weight. The weight loss is not *caused* by the product but rather by the diet. Yet millions of people continue to buy these expensive placebos and keep the companies in business.

Timing of a study is important. Two or more groups can only be validly compared if they are studied simultaneously. In other words, the study cannot first be conducted on one group, then the other group be studied at a later time. This can confound the study results in many ways, including change of climate, time of year, etc.

Parallel or crossover design refers to when and how study groups are exposed to study variables. Parallel design simply means that each of the study groups were studied at the same time, in the same fashion. For example, suppose we were going to study the effects of drug X over placebo. Drug X is a new drug, and most people with the condition had been taking drug Z coming into the study. In order to control for the effects of drug Z, patients are "washed out" for three weeks (taken off of drug Z) before being randomized to either drug X or placebo. The general study design diagram would look something like this:

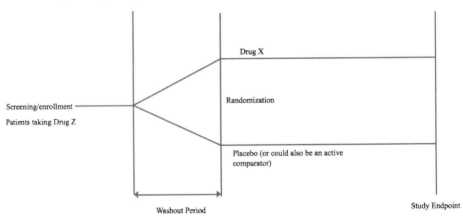

Parallel Study Design

Each group is studied for the same exact amount of time. There is also a number of study visits planned throughout, during which safety and efficacy parameters are assessed. The point is that the study is *prospective, randomized,* and *controlled.* Once the study is over, the raw data are collected—thousands and thousands of data points. The data are reviewed and interpreted by statisticians and other scientists in accordance to the stated, pre-planned analyses (called *a priori* definitions).

Crossover studies can be even better than parallel studies. However, they are considerably more expensive to conduct so are not as commonly done. The crossover study has all of the same controls as the parallel study design, but at some predefined time point, patients are switched, preferably in a blinded fashion, to the other treatment group. If each of the treatment groups experiences the same outcomes, the data are even more convincing than the parallel study design because there is a demonstrated *consistency* in the results. The illustrated diagram below depicts a *double*-crossover design, whereby patients are then put back on the original medication they received in the beginning. Using this study design demonstrates reproducibility of the initial study data even more strongly but comes with a much higher expense to conduct.

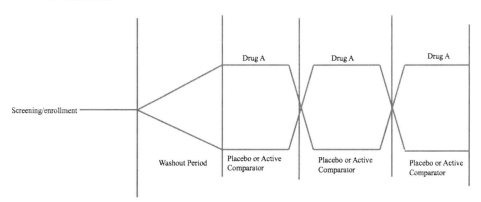

Double Crossover Study Design

The purpose of sharing this information with you is to highlight what type of work really goes into good science. So when you hear "clinical studies prove," put on your thinking cap, and remember what goes into the basics of good, valid scientific studies. This information merely scratches the surface of the world of clinical science, but should help you better discern the claims you may hear. There are many different types of studies out there, but the principles we discussed are the gold standards of good science. Studies that only look at a few patients, without any control group, lack the scientific rigor needed to fully interpret the results. The best approach is to really understand the science (if any) that is going behind the claims being made. If you don't understand what makes good science, you are much more likely to be misled.

Meta-analysis is an analytical technique in which the results of multiple studies are summarized.[1] By combining several similar studies' results the sample size is increased, which increases the powering of study effects, particularly in assessing the safety of a product. Meta-analyses can be extremely helpful if they are properly conducted. However, their results are sometimes questioned if the authors violated any of the fine critical principles in conducting a sound analysis. As you will see, meta-analyses of published studies from the pharmaceutical industry can be very limited due to the industry's withholding negative study results. I do tend to trust meta-analyses conducted in an academic setting more, particularly when there are no overt financial incentives for the published study results.

There are far too many examples of product claims versus available scientific data to list them all here. However, a safe general statement is that even the most commonly used herbal remedies have at best, conflicting study results; the claims themselves are not consistently reproducible. And as you will see in the next chapter, the U.S. government has hamstrung itself through legislation so that it does not have the same authority over the supplement industry as it does the pharmaceutical industry. Thus, there are many potential safety concerns that go unaddressed until a problem is identified *after* the product has been on the market for a period.

Another concern not routinely thought of is that many herbal remedies on the market have been found to be adulterated with unapproved drug substances, heavy metals, and other contaminants. In the United States, we really take for granted the safety of supplements and herbal remedies since the FDA helps to ensure the safety of our food and drugs. In the case of herbal remedies, we simply do not enjoy the same protection.

There are also questionable ethics in the scientific practices of pharmaceutical companies. For example, a particularly egregious practice is the fact that studies that turned out positive for a drug product are far more likely to be published than negative studies. This is called *publication bias*. We discussed this in the case of the negative study for Vytorin®, in which Merck® would not publish this study until a congressional inquiry began. There are many other examples of this. A good example was illustrated in an article that analyzed studies of antidepressants by looking at all of the studies on specific products that were registered with the FDA. It uncovered the fact that 97 percent of the positive studies were published, while only 12 percent of the negative studies were published.[2] When the negative studies were not published and not included in the overall analysis, the positive effects of the individual drugs increased anywhere from 11–69 percent and 32 percent overall! This practice then undermines the ability of practitioners to truly weigh the benefits versus the risks of a product because they have not seen all of the negative studies. Because of publication bias in the pharmaceutical industry, meta-analyses of drug studies have severe limitations because of the scarcity of the negative studies.

THE DIETARY SUPPLEMENT INDUSTRY: DOES THE GOVERNMENT PROTECT YOU?

Before we begin, we must first acknowledge that food, drug, and dietary supplement law is extremely complicated. If you want an in-depth look at these topics, there are several great authors and government agency websites that can answer any questions you may have. Our discussion here is a simplified version of these laws for you to keep in mind the next time you're at the drug store and you see a tempting "miracle" herb or supplement on the shelf.

The U.S. Food and Drug Administration (FDA) is the primary government agency responsible for regulating the safety of foods, drugs, cosmetics, and medical devices and the accuracy of statements made to promote those products. If the FDA finds a food to be adulterated because it has dangerous or unsanitary ingredients or was made in a factory that didn't follow Good Manufacturing Practices (GMPs) or is missing some essential ingredient, that adulterated food is generally taken off the market.[1] Foods can also be misbranded if a manufacturer gives it a false or misleading label or has other defects in the packaging or label. Misbranded foods are also subject to recall.

Drugs are far more heavily regulated than foods. In addition to having to meet similar cleanliness and branding regulations as foods, drugs also have to meet certain purity and strength standards and be proven safe and effective, usually through extensive clinical trials, before the FDA will allow them to be marketed.[2,3]

It generally takes between five and a half years to eleven years for a new drug to go from preclinical development (animal testing) through Phases I-III of clinical testing before it will make it to market.[4] During Phase I, a pharmaceutical company first tests how a drug works in the human body, either in healthy individuals or patients with the disease the drug is intended to treat. The company establishes how the drug is absorbed and metabolized, as well as probable effective dosages. In Phase II, the company tests the likelihood of the drug being effective in patients with the disease for which the drug is being investigated. In Phase III, the final phase to submit data to the FDA for approval, the company investigates the balance between the drug's safety and efficacy,[5] sometimes using other drugs as active comparators. This process amounts to tens of millions of dollars and potentially thousands of human test subjects, and a drug can *still* fail to make it to market. In this case, the drug company absorbs the financial loss. This, in part, helps to explain why drugs are so expensive; the companies must make up for the product's cost lost in the development process.

Before 1994, dietary supplements such as multivitamins and similar items that claimed to support health were regulated either like foods or drugs based primarily on the claims made to market them.[6] If a supplement was used for taste, aroma, or nutritive value, it was regulated as if it were food; if a supplement claimed to treat or prevent disease, it was regulated as if it were a drug.[7] Before 1994, there was quite a bit of struggling between supplement companies, the FDA, and congress. The FDA generally wanted greater power over supplements, while the supplement industry naturally wanted less regulation. Like most industries, the supplement industry had some good lobbyists and powerful allies intent on impacting how their products were regulated.

Enter Orrin Hatch, a republican senator from Utah. Senator Hatch was the driving force behind the Dietary Supplement Health and Education Act (DSHEA) of 1994, which opened the floodgates for poorly studied supplements to come to market. Utah's third largest industry is dietary supplements.[8] It is known as the "Silicon Valley" for dietary supplements, so it is no surprise that a politician from Utah introduced DSHEA. President Bill Clinton ratified the bill, making it truly a bipartisan disaster.

In the congressional findings for DSHEA, congress stated that in 1994, the United States would spend over $1 trillion for health care, and that by supporting the supplement industry, they believed that overall healthcare cost would decrease due to having a healthier population. However, this has not been the case. Today, the United States spends about $2.5 trillion for healthcare—more than twice the amount spent in 1994.[9] In addition, in 1994, the supplement industry grossed around $4 billion per year, but since DSHEA was passed, that amount has grown to over $25 Billion.[10, 11] But if these supplements were to create a healthier nation and we are spending more than six times the amount of money on supplements than we were in 1994, why did our overall healthcare costs go up? Could it be that the supplements that are on the market now as a result of DSHEA are in large part a load of snake oil and magic beans? While there are some supplements out there with good data to prove they are beneficial (multivitamins, omega-3 supplements, etc.), there are also many supplements that do not work or, even worse, have dangerous or otherwise unacceptable side effects.

DSHEA completely changed the way the FDA regulates dietary supplements. Instead of regulating supplements as either drugs or foods, DSHEA made supplements a special subset of food, which means that a drug-like dietary supplement no longer goes through the same premarket testing as drugs do before going to market. The testing standards for a supplement are now far lower than that of a medicine being studied for the same ailment.

Whereas a medicine for the treatment of a disease would have to go through preclinical trials and the three phases of clinical trials with large numbers of human test subjects, a supplement claiming to help with a disease can either provide scientific evidence or draw on statements by federal scientific bodies for support. This proof is better than nothing, but it is a far cry from the exacting standards the FDA applies to medicines. As you will see, proving health claims is fairly easy. There is a list of nutrients that the FDA accepts as having certain benefits (e.g., calcium deficiency is associated with osteoporosis, so a supplement containing calcium can claim to help reduce the risk of osteoporosis), whether or not that particular product has been tested in humans.[12] To take advantage of this listing, the label must qualify the claim with statements about the importance of calcium from a balanced diet; it cannot claim a certain percent of risk reduction, etc.[13]

Let's look a bit deeper at the calcium example, as it is a good clean example from which to illustrate how easy it is for the supplement industry to simply latch on to data not directly obtained from the product they are marketing. First, it is somewhat alarming that the rigorous three-phase testing isn't required even if the supplement claims to affect the structure or function of the body. In the case of calcium supplements, the labeling might state that the purpose of the product is to build strong bones, yet there are no data upon which to base that claim for that particular product. But because it is known that calcium is required in the building and maintenance of bone structure, that product can make a claim because it contains calcium. So unlike the credible scientific arena in which the product in question must demonstrate *itself* to possess the assumed trait, the product can hang on the coat tails of other scientific evidence, such as what might have been published by the USDA decades ago. The bottom line is that there is an unscientific leap in logic; how do you know if the product you are buying will build stronger bones in you? You really don't know because the product wasn't tested in patients fitting your personal description: your age, gender, health status. Now let's apply that same logic to a potential drug that could come to the market.

Suppose that there are solid scientific data (i.e., good science) that demonstrate a relationship between having enough estrogen in the body and the risk for miscarriages. Wouldn't it make sense, based on the logic used in the calcium example, that pregnant women might need to take estrogen to prevent miscarriages? From 1938 to 1971 the medical community did actually prescribe an estrogen called diethylstilbesterol (known as DES) for this very reason based on this very theory. The outcome of this belief was horrific. It turned out that women who took DES were then at an increased risk for developing breast cancer. Then, daughters of women who took DES (called DES daughters) began having problems with developing cervical and vaginal clear cell cancer, as well as fertility problems. DES sons have a higher rate of testicular cancer. Now being studied are the daughters and sons of DES daughters and DES sons—the DES third generation. While some questions still remain, it does appear that sons of DES daughters are twenty times more likely to have a displaced opening to the penis called hypospadias. (For more information on this, visit http://www.cdc.gov/des/consumers/about/concerns_offspring.html.) The point is that just because there may be an association between a certain disease state and a drug or dietary supplement, unless that product itself is rigorously tested, valid risk:benefit analyses cannot be conducted.

The case of the calcium supplement may seem extreme in terms of requiring that each calcium supplement product demonstrate that it fulfills the claim of building strong bone, but if you take that principle and apply it to other less-proven supplements, it becomes alarming in terms of the claims being made versus the actual scientific evidence. Then if you consider that many dietary supplements contain more than one herb or other component, you can hopefully see how the reduced oversight by the FDA of the supplement companies has become the disaster it has.

Note that a health claim is much different than a drug claim; drug claims state the product's ability to treat, prevent, cure, mitigate, or diagnose a disease. Only FDA-approved drugs and medical devices can make drug claims. Disease claims require either using one of the approved health claims or gaining official drug FDA approval.[14] Remember, while health claims may be watered-down versions of drug claims (such as claiming a dietary supplement supports good cholesterol levels), the layperson does not necessarily recognize the difference. Can you see just how tricky it is and how dietary supplements get away with making claims relative to diseases? And although any structure/function or disease claim must be tempered by adding to the label that the Food and Drug Administration has not evaluated the claims, most people don't let that stop them from buying the product from a slick salesperson. Fortunately, some companies are getting caught with their hands in the cookie jar; as of this writing, there is a class action lawsuit against the maker of a men's health daily vitamin for allegedly unsupported prostate cancer claims.

Dietary supplements are still subject to the rules regarding adulteration and misbranding, which means that if a supplement contains a dangerous substance (whether it is the supplement itself or is a contaminant), was made in an unsanitary manner, or is labeled in a way that is false or misleading, the FDA can take action against them. However, the FDA is stretched beyond its limits as it is with the pharmaceutical industry regulation. False and misleading statements from the dietary supplement industry are not likely to get top priority unless there are clear signals that a product has harmed many people.

Fortunately, dietary supplements are also subject to the Good Manufacturing Practices (GMPs) set by the FDA, the requirements of which are more stringent that those used for foods. GMPs generally help to regulate production, record keeping, and testing of supplements. Dietary supplement makers must also comply with the New Dietary Ingredients (NDI) provisions of DSHEA. The NDI provisions require a supplement maker to notify the FDA if they intend to market a dietary ingredient not previously marketed in the United States in a supplement before October 15, 1994. Under section 413(b) of the Food, Drug, and Cosmetic Act (21 U.S.C. 350b), a supplement containing an NDI will be deemed adulterated unless the ingredients have previously been in the food supply and are unchanged *or* if it fits the below statement:

> There is a history of use or other evidence of safety establishing that the dietary ingredient when used under the conditions recommended or suggested in the labeling of the dietary supplement will reasonably be expected to be safe and, at least 75 days before being introduced or delivered for introduction into interstate commerce, the manufacturer or distributor of the dietary ingredient or dietary supplement provides the FDA with information, including any citation to published articles, which is the basis upon which the manufacturer or distributor has concluded that a dietary supplement containing such dietary ingredient will reasonably be expected to be safe.

But there is a wrinkle to these rules. Under DSHEA, a supplement manufacturer is responsible for ensuring that their product is safe before it reaches the market. However, the NDI notification is just that: a *notification*. There is no requirement that the FDA approve the NDI before it goes to market, a company need only tell the FDA their intent to use the ingredients! The FDA can take action against an unsafe product after it reaches the market but only if it can demonstrate that the product or one of its components is unsafe. How does the FDA know that a supplement is unsafe? Manufacturers are now required to report to the FDA any adverse events that happened to people taking their supplements. Incredibly, it took thirteen years after the passage of DSHEA to make adverse event reporting mandatory! Until 2007, adverse event reporting was voluntary on the part of manufacturers[15]—the equivalent of the fox watching the henhouse. On top of all these barriers for the FDA to protect the public from dangerous supplements, DSHEA switched the burden of proof on to the FDA to prove that a supplement is *dangerous*. So again, unlike drug companies that have to prove to the FDA that their drugs are safe and effective, the FDA has to prove that a supplement is *not* safe in order to take it off the market. Given the limitations of funding and other resourcing, it is no wonder that more supplements aren't being removed from the market.

According to *Consumer Reports*, there are roughly 54,000 supplements listed in the Natural Medicines Comprehensive Database. DSHEA has allowed manufacturers to flood the marketplace with supplements as the FDA struggles to keep up. Of those 54,000, only about a third (18,000) of those supplements have safety and efficacy supported by science, and roughly 12 percent (6,480) are associated with dangerous side effects.[16]

Another important note is that many dietary supplements are stamped with what appears to be a formal approval from the *Homeopathic Pharmacopoeia of the United States*. You should know that does not mean that the product has been tested by some homeopathic agency for effectiveness and safety. The *Homeopathic Pharmacopoeia* is an encyclopedia of homeopathic products that was written before 1923, long before any legislation controlling the development and distribution of supplements was enacted. It certainly is not a valid stamp of approval.

Between 2008 and 2010, there were 170 voluntary recalls on supplements that illegally contained drugs or steroids.[17] Between June 2010 and September 2012, there were fifty-three supplements that were recalled, withdrawn, or subject to an FDA safety alert.[18] Most of those fifty-three had problems because they contained an "unapproved new drug" or "undeclared drug ingredients." Most of these were primarily used for sexual enhancement or weight loss.

In spite of the dangers posed by many supplements, the FDA to date has only successfully banned one supplement: ephedra. As we previously discussed, this ban took place in 2004. However, the FDA had been warning the public about the dangers of ephedra since 1997. Even after the ban, there was a drawn out legal battle between the industry and FDA, which the FDA ultimately won. Guess who had to pay for that legal battle? Of course, the public supports the FDA through tax dollars.

There are still many supplements on the shelves of drug stores that pose dangers (on top of being ineffective). There are also books and practitioners who recommend these products without clear knowledge of whether there is good science to prove its effectiveness and safety and sometimes without providing full disclosure about the potential negative consequences. For example, the Uva Ursi label contains a warning for people who already have kidney problems to avoid the supplement; however, it failed to warn that Uva Ursi could cause serious liver damage.[19] Similarly, the Kava Kava label warns against taking the supplement if you already have liver problems, but it has been associated with liver damage in at least thirty people in Europe, and it is unclear whether those cases were people with prior history of liver problems.[20] Kava Kava is banned in Germany, Canada, and Switzerland, and the FDA warned consumers about its dangers in 2002.[21] But because of the way the U.S. law is structured, Kava Kava is still on the market; the FDA cannot ban it without the same battle as occurred with ephedra.

Let's now turn our attention to a particularly egregious example of corporate greed. Colloidal silver (CS), which can be purchased at health food stores, has absolutely no warnings on the label. Colloidal silver consists of tiny particles of silver suspended in liquid that you can drink after mixing it with water. While supplement companies are careful to avoid claiming disease benefits, colloidal silver is purported on the Internet to help with infections, rosacea, HIV/AIDS, and a host of other conditions. The truth is that according to the National Institutes of Health:

> There is no scientific evidence for effectiveness and a severe risk for serious side effects from colloidal silver exists. The FDA does not consider colloidal silver to be safe or effective for treating any disease or condition and has issued an advisory regarding its safety.[22]

And that based on reviews of scientific literature,

> Silver has no known function in the body...Claims that there can be a "deficiency" of silver in the body and that such a deficiency can lead to disease are unfounded...Colloidal silver can have serious side effects.[23]

Colloidal silver (CS) is associated with neurological problems and kidney damage, but unlike many supplements that cause damage to the internal organs that is not outwardly visible, it can also cause damage that is visibly obvious. CS can actually turn skin a bluish-gray color, a condition called *argyria*. This color change is permanent (although some sufferers have been able to restore their skin color using expensive laser treatments).

In the 1950s, colloidal silver was a prescription drug; however, the FDA law at that time was less strict than it is now for drugs coming to the market. Rosemary Jacobs, a New York native, was prescribed nose drops containing colloidal silver at that time (although there was evidence of skin discoloration from CS since the 1930s). The inside of the nose consists of mucous membranes that allow for systemic absorption (the drug gets into the bloodstream from this route). Rosemary took those nose drops intermittently for three years, and at the age of fourteen, her skin had turned a slate-gray color.

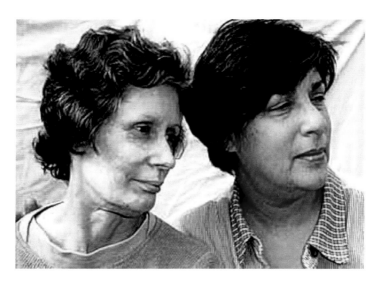

Silver (in the form of silver nitrate sticks and silver sulfadi-azine cream, not oral colloidal silver) is still used in hospitals legitimately for topical applications. These formulations of silver do not allow for systemic absorption as was observed with col-loidal silver. CS no longer exists as an FDA approved oral drug that physicians can prescribe, and the FDA banned it as an over-the-counter drug in 1999. Unfortunately though, it is still readily available in health food and other stores and online as a dietary supplement.[24] How can it be that the FDA can ban its use as a drug but not as a supplement? We can thank the DSHEA for the FDA's impotency in protecting the public safety. The dan-gers of colloidal silver are still present in these supplements, and Rosemary, among others, continues to speak out against supple-ment manufacturers who offer the product. Rosemary was kind enough to give us permission to use her picture in writing this chapter. Rosemary has her share of detractors on the internet, some claiming that she is a prop for the pharmaceutical industry against the supplement industry or that she's generally biased. However, as you can see, she clearly has a justifiable reason for taking up this crusade.

Comfrey root continues to be recommended to be taken orally through teas or infusions to treat lung problems and gastrointestinal symptoms. However, it contains liver damaging alkaloids, with the potential to cause liver failure. And while the FDA advised manufacturers to remove comfrey root in all products in 2001, it has not been banned. In fact, it is still being recommended for oral use and is still readily available to purchase online from American companies. This example illustrates why it is so important that you question any recommendation to use any herbal supplement; be sure to do your homework on it before taking it.

We've discussed the labels on these supplements, but what about commercials on TV and ads on the radio, internet, and in the newspaper—who regulates them, and how? Dietary supplements and nonprescription drug ads are regulated by the Federal Trade Commission (FTC), and the general requirement is that ads be truthful and not misleading and supported by substantial evidence before the ads can air.[25] On the other hand, prescription drug ads are regulated by the FDA and are subject to higher standards; legal prescription drug ads must have a fair balance between the drug's benefits and side effects or risks. It is almost comical to hear prescription drug ads on TV, for no sooner do they tell you how wonderful the drug is than you hear all of the bizarre potential side effects that can occur while taking the drug. The next time you are watching TV, see if you can compare the ads you see for FDA-approved drugs versus supplements; you will notice that the side effects and dangers of the drugs are much more prominent. It is not that the drug companies are just that honest; they are forced by the FDA to provide the litany of side effects observed in their clinical trials, whether or not those side effects were actually caused by the drug.

Keep in mind that "truthful and not misleading" is the standard for most ads, not just dietary supplements. But when was the last time you saw an ad for a product that did not live up to the

hype? Probably fairly recently. That's not to say that the FTC
doesn't keep some really misleading ads away from the public.
In fact, the FTC sometimes requires companies who have made
misleading statements to correct the misperception by making
disclaimers in future advertisements. For example, the FTC
recently required Bayer, the maker of Yaz® birth control pills,
to air corrective advertising on national television. Nevertheless,
even those misleading ads can make it to the public because the
FTC only regulates ads after they have been published—this
means that bad ads can get to the public and influence people
before the FTC has the chance to stop them.

Keep in mind that even if an ad conforms to FTC requirements, it doesn't mean that the product advertised is a good one.
Remember from earlier in the book that we mentioned a supplement whose studies were published in reputable medical journals,
but if you read the actual article, you would have seen that the
studies showed the supplement was not effective. The same idea
applies here. A one-thousand-year-old ancient Chinese remedy just needs to have come from China and been used for one
thousand years—it doesn't have to be safe and effective, proven
through valid scientific research.ˑ The FTC does what it can to
make sure that supplement companies do not use "weasel words"
to imply qualities or levels of support that are not accurate. In
its own words, the FTC looks at a number of factors in deciding
whether a supplement claim is substantiated, but the ultimate
decision is still subjective. The factors considered are as follows:

---

*   For further reading, check out "Dietary Supplements: An Advertising
    Guide For Industry" at http://business.ftc.gov/documents/bus09-
    dietary-supplements-advertising-guide-industry to learn more about
    the type of evidence required for supplement manufacturers to make
    claims such as scientists agree, etc.

The Type of Product

Generally, products related to consumer health or safety require a relatively high level of substantiation.

The Type of Claim

Claims that are difficult for consumers to assess on their own are held to a more exacting standard. Examples include health claims that may be subject to a placebo effect or technical claims that consumers cannot readily verify for themselves.

The Benefits of a Truthful Claim and the Cost/Feasibility of Developing Substantiation for the Claim

These factors are often weighed together to ensure that valuable product information is not withheld from consumers because the cost of developing substantiation is prohibitive. This does not mean, however, that an advertiser can make any claim it wishes without substantiation simply because the cost of research is too high.

The Consequences of a False Claim

This includes physical injury, for example, if a consumer relies on an unsubstantiated claim about the therapeutic benefit of a product and foregoes a proven treatment. Economic injury is also considered.

The Amount of Substantiation that Experts in the Field Believe is Reasonable

In making this determination, the FTC gives great weight to accepted norms in the relevant fields of research and consults with experts from a wide variety of disciplines, including those with experience in botanicals and traditional medicines. Where there is an existing standard for substantiation developed by a government agency or other authoritative body, the FTC accords great deference to that standard.[26]

Just keep in mind what you now know about valid scientific studies; purchase only those items that can meet the gold standard principles. Know without a doubt what is going into your body. It is the only body you have, after all, so why risk damaging it based on unsubstantiated claims? Remember that supplements, unlike medicines, do not have to be tested for efficacy before going to market. Supplement makers are responsible for making supplements safe before they go on the market—the FDA only takes action *after* people are already exposed to danger. Even if a supplement is not dangerous, it isn't necessarily effective. So think before spending your hard-earned money on a supplement that claims to have the miraculous ability to melt pounds without you changing your lifestyle or something similar. If it sounds too good to be true, it probably is.

DIET, SUPPLEMENTS, AND YOUR PRESCRIPTION AND OVER-THE-COUNTER MEDICATION

· ·

To round out our discussion about becoming your own scientist, let's consider the total picture of what you put into your body on a daily basis. To say that there are far too many medicines, supplements and foods to keep track of all of the potential interactions is a gross understatement. While many of these interactions are fairly well known, it is likely that many more have not yet been identified. In that we can only work with the information available, we will never get it all perfect. However, because of the possible combinations and the unlikelihood that all potential interactions will be spotted by your healthcare provider(s), it is of utmost importance that you stay on top of everything you take and how it may interact with other drugs, supplements, and foods.

There are many different mechanisms that can cause interactions between drugs, supplements, and diet. Briefly, some of the main reasons for interactions include:

- Direct binding of substances, preventing absorption of one of them—A good example of this is when ciprofloxacin, an antibiotic, is taken within two hours with magnesium-containing antacids. The antacid binds to the ciprofloxacin, preventing it from being absorbed into the bloodstream. This can reduce the effectiveness of the antibiotic.

• Blocking of enzymes that normally break drugs down— Grapefruit juice is known to interact with many drugs in this manner, including statins, some blood pressure drugs, and some antidepressants. Since the breakdown of the drugs is being prevented, blood levels of the drugs rise. This makes it more likely that you would experience side effects associated with the drug, and in severe cases, the drug levels can become toxic.

• Competing for the same enzyme for metabolism— Zocor®, a statin, and diltiazem, a blood pressure medication, compete for the same enzyme for metabolism. The result can be an increased blood level of one or both medications, leading to potentially dangerous side effects. However, a positive effect of this type of interaction is that because of the lower metabolism of one or both drugs, you may actually be able to reduce the dosage of either or both. This type of interaction is actually used clinically. A drug called probenecid, which is used to prevent elevated level of uric acid (which can lead to gout), inhibits the metabolism of penicillin. It is often used together with penicillin in patients with gonorrhea to keep the blood level of penicillin high in order to more effectively treat it.

This drug interaction can also be dangerous. For example, a drug called tramadol, used for pain, can compete with any other drug that is also metabolized by the enzymes CYP2D6 and CYP3A4 and vice versa. I recently saw a devastating interaction between tramadol and aripiprazole, a drug that was being used as an adjunct therapy to treat major depressive disorder in a patient. The patient began to suffer from a condition called tardive dyskinesia, which is in most cases a permanent movement disorder. The patient's head started shaking uncontrollably, and he could not keep one of his eyes opened. There is no cure per se for tardive dyskinesia; this patient will suffer from this for the rest of his life, all due to this drug interaction.

- Enzyme induction—Some medications can increase the activity of enzymes that metabolize another medication, resulting in decreased effectiveness of the second medication. For example, some antibiotics induce the enzymes that metabolize birth control pills (BCPs). This can decrease the effectiveness of the BCP, potentially allowing for an unwanted pregnancy.

- Protein binding—Some medications, such as phenytoin sodium (used in epilepsy), are bound to protein in the blood stream. If another medication or substance is taken that is more tightly bound to protein, it can push the phenytoin off of the protein molecule, thereby increasing the blood level of phenytoin. Higher blood levels can lead to more unwanted side effects of phenytoin, such as slurred speech, slowed movement, and confusion.

- Direct competition—Warfarin, a medicine used as an anticoagulant to prevent heart attacks, strokes, and pulmonary emboli (clots in the lungs), works by directly inhibiting the action of vitamin K, a procoagulant. If one increases his/her vitamin K intake from their established norm upon which the warfarin was titrated for optimal anticoagulation (usually by increasing their intake of leafy green vegetables significantly), the effectiveness of the warfarin can be greatly decreased, increasing the patient's risk for these cardiovascular events.

What if you discover that one or more medicines you take interact with each other? Some of these are absolutely unavoidable in some medical conditions; you just need to be aware of warning signals that there is a serious problem. Take care to ensure that all health care providers you see know about all of the medications and dietary supplements you take. I also recommend you have all of your prescriptions filled at the same pharmacy so that your pharmacist can also spot problems before they occur.

Many interactions are avoidable, however, through a change in medication or diet. For example, if you are prescribed a medicine for high cholesterol and it interacts with a medicine being used to lower your blood pressure, it is likely that there is another medication in the same class of either of these medications that will not have the same interaction. Another example is with MAO inhibitors used for severe depression. It is known that foods containing tyromine (some wines, fermented cheeses, and cured meats) can interact with these medicines, potentially causing a hypertensive crisis that could lead to death. This interaction potential exists for up to a month after the drug is discontinued. A well-educated consumer can easily avoid the interaction by avoiding tyromine-containing foods.

Interactions between drugs and dietary supplements can be every bit as unpleasant and dangerous as drug-drug interactions. For example, St. John's Wort can decrease the effectiveness of birth control pills through enzyme induction, just like some antibiotics, potentially allowing for an unwanted pregnancy. It can also decrease the effectiveness of drugs used after an organ transplant to prevent rejection, as well as reduce the effectiveness of some HIV medications.

The point of this discussion is simply to make you aware that almost nothing you take is completely innocuous; everything has a potential to affect how you feel as well as your well being. You need to be mindful that harmful interactions can occur between various substances you put into your body, including foods and supplements. You need to know what all of the safety issues are of all medications and dietary supplements you take, as well as how they interact with certain foods. And before you make any changes to medications you are already taking, be sure to discuss them with your physician.

SOME FINAL COMMENTS

· ·

We have taken quite a journey together in this book. You now know how to become 95% vegan, assess your basic health and nutritional status, maintain adequate intake of protein, which fats to include (and quantities), how to make veganism work for you in a number of medical conditions, how to lose weight with a vegan diet, and the importance of and how to assess the claims made by the pharmaceutical and dietary supplement industries. You have completed all of the Homeworks, so you should feel very prepared to move forward and begin your healthier life.

If at any time you have slipped or completely fallen off the wagon, you can always come back to this book for a refresher. At the same time, I strongly encourage you to try to stay abreast of new/updated scientific information but with a critical eye on whether it is *good* science.

Please continue to strive for good health through your daily nutritional decisions. But always remember, you do not have to be *perfect* to be highly *successful*! Don't ever judge your value by how good you are on your diet. Also, don't judge your value by your weight, blood sugar, or blood pressure. It always amazes me how some people beat themselves up for the most minor imperfections.

On the other hand, there are those people who continue to make excuses and delude themselves into believing they are exempt from the ultimate health outcomes. Life is truly fragile, and your health is more important than anything. There are certainly many affluent people with cancer who say they would give up all of their riches for good health. Treat your body as the amazing gift it is. You only get one.

If you read this book because you already have a chronic disease you are trying to control better through nutrition, hats off to you for your perseverance! Always remember that it is very worth your time to continue to try to keep your illness from progressing. There are many people on dialysis who wish they had paid closer attention to their blood pressure and/or blood sugar control. Don't ever give up on yourself or your health!

As the saying goes, "Desperate people do desperate things." I see this often when people feel out of control with their eating habits, typically when they are overweight. This mindset causes them to give up favorite foods, try fad diets, and cut their caloric intake by extremes. I hope that by reading this book, you have come to realize that this is not a prudent way to go. By focusing on having proper nutrition and the caloric intake to match the weight you want to attain, you will be amazingly successful and wonder why you ever tried any other route.

Most importantly, please do not forget that you need to understand what your target goals are for blood pressure, cholesterol, BMI, weight, etc. Remember, even the best marksman cannot hit the target if he or she cannot *see* the target. All of your targets should have been written down or otherwise recorded in your Homework assignments. If you are doing the best you can and are still not achieving your target, do not hesitate to seek help from your physician. It is *critical* that you achieve and maintain these targets to avoid bad outcomes.

And finally, we wish you the very best in your life journey. We wish you good physical and mental health. We wish it for your families and your future generations. It is up to you to create the ripple effect. You have the tools to do so; may you always have the wisdom and commitment to carry it out.

APPENDIX 1

· ·

SUGGESTED RESOURCES

Books/Cookbooks:

Moskowitz, Isa Chandra. *Appetite for Reduction.* Da Capo Press: 2011.

Schinner, Miyoko. *Artisan Vegan Cheese.* Book Publishing Company: 2012.

Davis, Brenda and Vesanto Melina. *Becoming Raw.* Book Publishing Company: 2010.

Andoh, Elizabeth. *Celebrating Japan's Vegan and Vegetarian Traditions, Kansha.* Ten Speed Press: 2010.

Schinner, Miyoko Nishimoto. *Japanese Cooking, Contemporary and Traditional, Simple, Delicious. and Vegan.* Book Publishing Company: 1999.

Olson, Cathe. *Lick It: Creamy, Dreamy Vegan Ice Creams Your Mouth Will Love.* Book Publishing Company: 2009.

Simpson, Alicia C. *Quick and Easy Low-Cal Vegan Comfort Food.* The Experiment: 2012.

Reinfeld, Mark and Jennifer Murray. *The 30 Minute Vegan*. Da Capo Press.

Savona, Natalie. *The Big Book of Juices*. Duncan Baird Publishers, Ltd, 2009.

Steen, Celine and Joni Marie Newman. *The Complete Guide to Vegan Food Substitutions*. Fair Winds Press, 2011.

Nixon, Lindsay S. *The Happy Herbivore*. Ben Bella Books, 2011.

Patrick-Goudreau, Colleen. *The Joy of Vegan Baking*. Fair Winds Press, 2007.

Bates, Dorothy R. *The TVP Cookbook*. Book Publishing Company, 1991.

Stepaniak, Jo. *The Ultimate Uncheese Cookbook*. Book Publishing Company, 2003.

Hester, Kathy. *The Vegan Slow Cooker*. Fair Winds Press, 2011.

Patrick-Goudreau, Colleen. *The Vegan Table*. Fair Winds Press, 2009.

Moskowitz, Isa Chandra and Terry Hope Romero. *Veganomicon*, Da Capo Press Lifelong Books, 2007.

Moskowitz, Isa Chandra. *Vegan Brunch*. Da Capo Press, 2009.

Simpson, Alicia C. *Vegan Celebrations*. The Experiment Publishing Company, 2010.

Simpson, Alicia C. *Vegan Comfort Food*. The Experiment, LLC, 2009.

Moskowitz, Isa Chandra and Terry Hope Romero. *Vegan Cookies Invade Your Cookie Jar*, Da Capo Press Lifelong Books, 2009.

Moskowitz, Isa Chandra and Terry Hope Romero. *Vegan Cupcakes Take Over the World*. Da Capo Press Lifelong Books, 2006.

Robertson, Robin. *Vegan on the Cheap*. John Wiley and Sons, Inc, 2010.

Moskowitz, Isa Chandra and Terry Hope Romero. *Vegan Pie in the Sky*. Da Capo Press Lifelong Books, 2011.

Stepaniak, Joanne. *Vegan Deli, Wholesome Ethnic Fast Food*, Book Publishing Company, 2011.

Hasson, Julie. *Vegan Diner*. Running Press Book Publishers, 2011.

Terry, Bryant. *Vegan Soul Kitchen*. Da Capo Press, 2009.

Stepaniak, Jo. *Vegan Vittles*. Book Publishing Company, 2007.

Web sites:

"Power Plate: Physicians Committee for Responsible Medicine." http://PCRM.org/health/powerplate

"Veganism in a Nutshell—The Vegetarian Resource Group." http://www.vrg.org/nutshell/vegan.htm#common

"My Net Diary." http://www.mynetdiary.com/

"National Diabetes Education Program." http://ndep.nih.gov

Diabetes Prevention Program: http://diabetes.niddk.nih.gov/dm/pubs/preventionprogram.

UKPDS Risk Tool: http://www.dtu.ox.ac.uk/riskengine/download.php

APPENDIX 2

• •

CITED RECIPES REPRINTED
WITH PERMISSION

Seitan Cutlets

Reprinted with permission from *Veganomicon* by Isa Chandra
Moskowitz and Terry Hope Romero. pg 132, published by Da
Capo Press, a member of the Perseus Books Group. Copyright©
2007.

Makes 6 cutlets

Broth:
    6 cups vegetable broth
    3 Tbsp. soy sauce
Cutlets:
    1-¼ cup vital wheat gluten
    ½ cup cold vegetable broth
    ¼ cup soy sauce
    1 Tbsp. olive oil
    2 cloves garlic, pressed or grated on a microplane grater
    1 tsp. grated lemon zest (optional)
Preheat the oven to 350° F.

Prepare the broth:

Bring to a boil in a pot and then turn off the heat and keep covered.

Prepare the cutlets:

Place the wheat gluten in a mixing bowl. Pour the cold vegetable broth (not the vegetable broth you brought to a boil, but the broth in the cutlet ingredients) into a measuring cup. Then pour in the soy sauce. Add the oil, garlic, and lemon zest and mix. Pour the wet mixture into the flour and combine with a wooden spoon until most of the moisture has absorbed and it's partially clumped up with the flour. Use your hands to knead for about three minutes until the dough is elastic. Divide into six equal pieces; the best way to do this is to roll it out into somewhat of a log shape and then slice it with a knife.

Take each piece and stretch and knead it into an oblong cutlet shape that is a little less than ½ inch thick. Use your body weight to press it and stretch it on a hard surface; there will be some resistance, but just keep at it.

Pour the heated vegetable broth into a 9 × 13–inch glass baking pan or a ceramic casserole (if all you have is metal, that is okay). Place the cutlets in the broth, then bake for about 30 minutes, uncovered, turn the cutlets over (use tongs for this for ease), and bake for an additional 20 minutes.

Remove from the oven and place the cutlets into a colander to drain. The cutlets are now ready to use in whatever seitan recipe you choose. If you have extra seitan, store it in the cooking liquid in a tightly covered container.

Southwest Tofu Scramble

Reprinted with permission from *The 30 Minute Vegan* by Mark Reinfeld and Jennifer Murray., pp 62-63, published by Da Capo Press, a member of the Perseus Books Group. Copyright© 2009.

Makes 4 servings

1-½ Tbsp. safflower oil
1 cup yellow onion, chopped small
1 small red bell pepper, seeded and minced
1 medium-sized jalapeño or other chile pepper, seeded and minced
4 medium-sized garlic cloves, pressed or minced
1 pound extra-firm tofu, crumbled into large chunks
¾ tsp. powdered turmeric
¾ tsp. paprika
3 Tbsp. nutritional yeast flakes
1-½ tsp. soy sauce or to taste
2 Tbsp. minced fresh cilantro
1-½ tsp. chile powder
1 tsp. ground cumin
½ cup salsa and/or corn kernels (optional)
Sea salt and black pepper

1. Place oil in a large sauté pan over medium-high heat. Add the onion, red bell pepper, jalapeño, and garlic and cook until the onion is soft, for about 3 minutes, stirring frequently.

2. Add the tofu. Cook for 5 minutes, stirring frequently.

3. Add the remaining ingredients, cook 3–5 minutes more, season to taste and enjoy.

Tempeh Bacon Revamped

Reprinted with permission from *Vegan Brunch* by Isa Chandra Moskowitz., pg 141, Published by Da Capo Press, a member of the Perseus Books Group. Copyright© 2009.

Serves 6–8 as a side

For the marinade:

3 Tbsp. soy sauce
1 Tbsp. liquid smoke
1 Tbsp. pure maple syrup
1 Tbsp. apple cider vinegar
1 Tbsp. olive oil
1 Tbsp. tomato paste
¾ cup vegetable broth
2 garlic cloves, crushed

To cook:

Cut widthwise into ¼-inch slices the 8–12 oz tempeh.
In a wide shallow bowl, mix together all the marinade ingredients. Add the tempeh slices and marinate them for about an hour.
Preheat a large, heavy-bottomed pan over medium heat. Panfry the tempeh in oil for about 7 minutes, flipping occasionally and adding more marinade as you flip. That's it!

Oatmeal Raisin Cookies

Reprinted with permission from *Vegan Cookies Invade Your Cookie Jar* by Isa Chandra Moskowitz and Terry Hope Romero, pg 75, published by Da Capo Press, a member of the Perseus Books Group. Copyright© 2009.

Makes 2 dozen cookies

1/3 cup soy milk
2 Tbsp. ground flax seeds
2/3 cup brown sugar
1/3 cup oil
1 tsp. pure vanilla extract
¾ cup flour

½ tsp. ground cinnamon
1/8 tsp. ground nutmeg
¼ tsp. baking soda
¼ tsp. salt
1 ½ cup quick-cooking oats
½ cup raisins

1. Preheat oven to 350° F. Line two baking sheets with parchment paper.

2. In a large bowl, use a fork to vigorously mix together the soymilk and flaxseeds. Add in the sugar and oil, and mix until it resembles caramel, about 2 minutes. Mix in the vanilla. Sift in the flour, spices, and salt, mixing the dry ingredients as they are being added. Fold in the oatmeal and raisins.

3. Drop dough in generous tablespoons, about 2 inches apart, onto the baking sheets. Flatten the tops a bit since they don't spread much. Bake for 10–12 minutes.

Old-Fashioned Rice Pudding

Reprinted with permission from *The Vegan Diner* by Julie Hasson. Available from Running Press, an imprint of The Perseus Books Group. Copyright © 2011.

Makes 4 to 6 Servings

1 cup medium-grain sushi rice
½ cup raisins, optional
1-½ to 2 cups soy milk or almond milk (plain or vanilla) or as needed
1 tsp. pure vanilla extract
freshly ground cinnamon

In a large saucepan over medium heat, combine 2 cups water, rice, and raisins (if using), and bring to a boil. Reduce heat to low, cover and simmer for 15 minutes.

Remove saucepan from heat and let sit, covered for 5 minutes. Remove the cover.

Add 1 cup of the soymilk and sugar to the cooked rice, stirring until combined. Return the saucepan to stove. Cook over medium heat, stirring often. Continue adding more milk as the pudding cooks and thickens, stirring as needed. Cook for 15 to 20 minutes, or until the pudding is very thick and creamy. If the pudding is too thick, stir in a little more soymilk as needed to thin slightly. Remove the saucepan from the heat and stir in the vanilla. Scoop the pudding into serving dishes and sprinkle with ground cinnamon. Refrigerate pudding until ready to serve.

Melty White Cheez

The Ultimate Uncheese Cookbook by Jo Stepaniak., Book Publishing Company, 2003. Used with permission by the author.

Makes 5 (¼ cup) servings

1-½ cups water or plain nondairy milk
¼ cup nutritional yeast flakes
¼ cup flour (any kind; your choice)
2 Tbsp. sesame tahini
2 Tbsp. kuzu, arrowroot, or cornstarch
2 Tbsp. fresh lemon juice
1 tsp. onion powder
¾ tsp. salt
¼ tsp. garlic powder

Place all ingredients in a blender and process until completely smooth. Transfer to a small saucepan. Cook over medium-high heat, stirring almost constantly with a wire whisk until very thick and smooth. Serve hot.

APPENDIX 3

HOW TO CALCULATE YOUR PERCENT [%] FAT INTAKE BY HAND*

See the chart on the following page.

A	B	C	D	E	F	G	H	I	J
Food Eaten	Calories per Portion Size	Portion Size	How Much You Ate (Use the Same Unit of Measure as for Portion Size)	Multiplier for Calculations (Divide Column D by Column C)	Total Calories (Multiply Column B and Column E)	Grams of Fat per Portion Size	Total Grams of Fat (Multiply Column G and Column E)	Total Calories from Fat (Multiply Column H by 9)	Percent (%) Calories from Fat (Divide Column I by Column F, Then Multiply by 100)
Sample Food A	100	1 Cup	1.25 Cups	1.25	125	2	2.5	23	18.0%
Sample Food B	450	4 oz	4 oz	1	450	10	10	90	20.0%
Sample Food C	80	15 small	20 small	1.33	106	0	0	0	0.0%
Day's Totals					681		12.5	113	16.6%

APPENDIX 4

TRACKING YOUR HEALTH STATUS

Please see the chart on the following pages.

	Target Goal	Date	Meaurement	Normal, Low or High (N, L, H)	Date	Meaurement	Normal, Low or High (N, L, H)
BMI							
Waist Circumference							
Blood Pressure							
Hemoglobin							
Hematocrit							
Serum Creatinine*							
Creatinine Clearance	>60 ml/min						
Liver Function Tests	Normal						
HDL							
LDL							
Triglycerides							
Blood Glucose							
Albumin Level							
Any Signs of Macrocytic Anemia?	NO						
TSH							
Vitamin D Level							
CRP Level							

* Please be sure to know what your creatinine clearance is - see http://www.globalrph.com/crcl.htm.

APPENDIX 5

• •

ORIGINAL RECIPES

High Protein Skillet Biscuit

Makes 12 ample servings

Use a 10-inch cast iron skillet. Skillet must be oven safe. If you do not have one, a 9 × 12-inch baking pan will do. Grease the skillet or pan, and set aside.

Ingredients:
1 24-oz package organic firm tofu (may substitute with 2 15-oz cans white beans)
1 large onion, chopped fine
3 cloves minced garlic
1 Tbsp. canola oil (can also use flax or olive)
¾ cup plain, light soymilk
10 oz frozen spinach, cooked per directions (may substitute with 10 oz frozen broccoli)
¼ cup nutritional yeast flakes
¼ teaspoon white pepper
1 tsp. salt (more or less, according to taste, if desired)
¼ tsp. turmeric
¼ tsp. nutmeg
2-½ cups self-rising flour

Preheat oven to 350°F. Heat oil in a medium skillet. When hot, sauté onion until tender. Set aside.

Place remaining ingredients, except for self-rising flour in blender. Process until completely smooth, scraping down sides as needed. Add onion and process for another 30 seconds. Pour mixture into large bowl. Add self-rising flour, and stir in well (may add more flour if the batter is too wet, but add in ¼ cup at a time, so as not to make the batter too dry).

Pour batter into greased skillet, and bake in oven for 30 minutes.

Per serving:
Calories: 163
Fat (gm): 3
Carbohydrate (gm): 24
Protein (gm): 9
Fiber (gm): 3

95% Vegan Food Choices™:
1 legume
½ grain

95% Vegan BUCs™: 2.25

Vegan Mexicali TVP Ground Beef

Makes 4 ample servings

This is a delicious substitute for ground beef in any Mexican recipe. TVP has a texture that is remarkably similar to ground beef, and with the right spices, it makes a wonderful burrito!

2 cups TVP (Texturized Vegetable Protein)
1-¾ cup boiling water
2 Tbsp. flaxseed oil
½ cup onion, diced

2 cloves garlic minced
½ Tbsp. cumin, or more to taste
2 Tbsp. soy sauce
1 tsp. salt

Combine TVP and boiling water; set aside while it puffs up.
Put flaxseed oil in a large skillet over medium heat, add onions and garlic, and sauté.
Add TVP mixture and remaining ingredients to skillet, combine, and cook until well-mixed and heated through.

Per Serving:
Calories: 235
Fat (gm): 8
Carbohydrate (gm): 17
Protein (gm): 25
Fiber (gm): 10

95% Vegan Food Choices™:
1.5 legumes
1 fat

95% Vegan BUCs™: 2.5

Vegan Italian TVP Ground Beef

Makes 4 ample servings

This is essentially an Italian version of the Mexicali TVP above; you may add it to a marinara sauce to make it meaty and replace either meatballs or meat sauce.

2 cups TVP (texturized vegetable protein)
1-¾ cup boiling water

2 Tbsp. flaxseed oil
½ cup onion, diced
2 cloves garlic minced
0.5 Tbsp. oregano (or more, to taste)
2 Tbsp. soy sauce
1 tsp. salt

Combine TVP and boiling water; set aside while it puffs up.

Put flaxseed oil in a large skillet over medium heat, add onions and garlic, and sauté.

Add TVP mixture and remaining ingredients to skillet, combine, and cook until well-mixed and heated through. Now you can add the Italian TVP to any pasta sauce for a high protein pasta dinner!

Per Serving:
Calories: 235
Fat (gm): 8
Carbohydrate (gm): 17
Protein (gm): 25
Fiber (gm): 10

95% Vegan Food Choices™:
1.5 legume
1 fat

95% Vegan BUCs™: 2.5

Chick'n Seitan

Makes 1 pound, roughly 5–3 oz servings

Seitan mixture:

1 cup vital wheat gluten

¼ cup nutritional yeast flakes
½ cup Better Than Bouillon® No Chicken Base prepared broth
(½ tsp. bouillon in ½ cup water)
¼ cup soy sauce
1 Tbsp. flax oil
1 Tbsp. minced or granulated garlic

Broth for cooking:

6 cups Better Than Bouillon® No Chicken Base prepared broth
(6 tsp. bouillon in 6 cups water)
¼ cup soy sauce

First combine the ingredients for the broth in a large sauce-pan, and begin cooking over high heat.

While the broth is coming to a boil, combine the seitan mixture ingredients in a separate bowl. Mix until completely blended, kneading if necessary. Add the seitan mixture to the boiling broth, and boil for 10 minutes. Reduce and let simmer for 30 minutes. Remove the seitan from the broth and slice into 3-oz portions (or larger if desired; however, calories are based on a 3-oz portion). Note that the protein from the vital wheat gluten is complemented by the lysine in the soy sauce and nutritional yeast flakes.

Per 3 oz Serving:
Calories: 180
Fat (gm): 5.5
Carbohydrate (gm): 15
Protein (gm): 48
Fiber (gm): 2

95% Vegan Food Choices™:
0.75 legume

1 grain

95% Vegan BUCs™: 2.5

Vegan Spritz Cookies

Makes 70 cookies

3-¾ cups whole wheat pastry flour (or you may use all-purpose flour)
1-½ cups Earth Balance® Vegan Buttery Sticks
¾ cup granulated sugar
¼ cup orange juice or apple juice
1 Tbsp. flaxseed meal, beaten together with 3 Tbsp. water (or
other egg replacement for 1 large egg)

Preheat oven to 350°F
In a large bowl, cream together the buttery sticks and sugar.
Next add the flaxseed mixture or other preferred egg replace-
ment, and the juice.
Slowly mix in the flour, and combine without over-mixing.
You can use either a cookie press or simply spoon tablespoons
of batter onto an ungreased cookie sheet.
If you want to decorate the cookies with sprinkles or colored
sugar, do it before baking; otherwise, the decorations will not stick.
Bake 8–10 minutes or until golden-brown.

Per Serving (1 cookie):
Calories: 67
Fat (gm): 4
Carbohydrate (gm): 7
Protein (gm): 0.7
Fiber (gm): 1

95% Vegan Food Choices™:

0.5 grain
0.25 fat

95% Vegan BUCs™: 1

Tofu Omelet

Serves 2–4; nutrition based on a 2 serving portion.

1 Tbsp. flaxseed oil
16 oz soft silken tofu
½ cup all-purpose flour
1 cup frozen spinach
½ cup green onions
2 cloves garlic, minced
4 oz. vegan cheddar cheese
Salt to taste

Optional: Sprinkle nutritional yeast flakes inside the omelet for a cheesier taste and an increase in protein, if desired.

Add oil to skillet over high heat, add green onions and spinach, and sauté.

While the greens are heating, combine tofu, flour, and garlic in a blender, and blend until creamy.

Add the tofu mixture over the greens and lower to medium heat. With a spatula, scramble the mixture, and leave to cook for 5 minutes. Repeat scrambling and letting the mixture cook until thick. Because there is tofu in this recipe, the omelet will never fully solidify. However it will thicken to the point that you can flip it with a spatula—flip it and spread the vegan cheese over the top of the omelet. Scramble it a little more to mix the cheese into the omelet. Serve while hot, adding salt and pepper to taste.

Per serving:
Calories: 570

Fat (gm): 31
Carbohydrate (gm): 48
Protein (gm): 29
Fiber (gm): 8

95% Vegan Food Choices™:
3 legumes
1 grain
1 vegetable
2 fat

95% Vegan BUCs™:
8.25

Easy Vegan Pizza

Makes 4 large slices (roughly equal to 2 slices from a large delivery pizzeria)

1 package pre-prepared pizza dough
1 24 oz jar marinara sauce
1 8 oz package of vegan mozzarella cheese, shredded
1 package frozen tri-colored peppers (or whatever vegetables you prefer)
Optional: Sprinkle nutritional yeast flakes on top for a cheesier taste and an increase in protein, if desired.

Preheat oven to 350°F

Sprinkle flour over a cookie sheet. Roll out dough over the flour. Bake the dough for 8 minutes, remove from oven, and let cool.

Spread marinara sauce, cheese, and vegetables over the crust, and bake for 10-15 minutes until cheese is melted and vegetables are hot.

Cut into 4 pieces and serve while hot.

Per serving (1/4 pizza):
Calories: 620
Fat (gm): 24
Carbohydrate (gm): 84
Protein (gm): 15
Fiber (gm): 7

95% Vegan Food Choices™:
4 grain
3 vegetable
2 fat

95% Vegan BUCs™: 8.25

Quick and Easy Vegan Pancakes

Makes 5 servings

2 cups Heart Healthy Bisquick®
1 Tbsp. ground flaxseed meal, beaten together with 3 Tbsp. water
1-¼ light soy milk

Blend ingredients, spoon out desired pancake batter, and cook in skillet over medium heat. Once edges of pancakes are solid, flip and let finish cooking.

While this recipe was made with Bisquick®, you can easily make your own pancake mix with 2 cups of all-purpose flour, 2 teaspoons baking powder, and 1 tsp. baking soda. We generally prefer to go the less-refined route with our foods, but the occasional packaged ingredient is fine.

Per serving:
Calories: 190

Fat (gm): 4
Carbohydrate (gm): 34
Protein (gm): 5
Fiber (gm): 1.6

95% Vegan Food Choices™:
2 grain

95% Vegan BUCs™: 3

Vegan Beef Stew

Makes 4 generous servings

4 cups vegetable broth *or* Better Than Bouillon® No Beef Base (4 tsp. in 4 cups hot water)
1 can kidney beans, drained and rinsed
½ lb carrots, sliced
1 can diced tomatoes or 5 diced fresh tomatoes
½ lb celery, sliced
1 large onion, diced
4 cloves garlic, minced

Combine ingredients in a Crock-Pot®, and allow to cook on low setting 5–8 hours. Alternatively combine ingredients in a large stockpot and cook over medium-high heat until the vegetables are tender.

Per Serving:
Calories: 155
Fat (gm): 0.5
Carbohydrate (gm): 32
Protein (gm): 7

Fiber (gm): 12

95% Vegan Food Choices™:
1 legumes
2 vegetable

95% Vegan BUCs™: 2

Vegan Corned Beef

Makes 1 medium loaf, 6 servings

Ingredients:
½ cup chickpeas
1 Tbsp. flaxseed oil
1 cup Better Than Bouillon® No Beef Base (1 tsp. bouillon combined with 1 cup hot water)
2 tsp. granulated garlic
1 tsp. salt
1 Tbsp. paprika
1 tsp. cloves
1 tsp. allspice
2 tsp. dried mustard
1-¼ cups vital wheat gluten

Start a large pot of water with a steamer basket over high heat. Combine all ingredients except vital wheat gluten in a blender, and blend until smooth. In a medium bowl, measure out 1-¼ cup vital wheat gluten. Pour the blended mixture over the gluten, and stir with a spoon until combined. Then knead by hand until it is a smooth ball of dough. Place on a large piece of aluminum foil, roll foil up, and make sure the edges are well-sealed. Steam in steamer basket for 1 hour. Let cool, slice, and serve.

Per serving:

Calories: 145
Fat (gm): 3
Carbohydrate (gm): 8
Protein (gm): 20
Fiber (gm): 2

95% Vegan Food Choices™:
1-½ grain

95% Vegan BUCs™: 2

Irish Soda Bread

One 9 × 5 inch loaf

Ingredients:
3 cups all-purpose flour
1 Tbsp. baking powder
1/3 cups white sugar
1 tsp. salt
1 tsp. baking soda
1 Tbsp. ground flaxseed mixed with 3 Tbsp. water
¼ cup Earth Balance® vegan butter, melted
2 cups vegan buttermilk (using a 2-cup measuring cup, add 4 Tbsp. white vinegar, and then fill the measuring cup up to the 2-cup line with plain soy milk. Set aside for a few minutes to curdle.)

Preheat oven to 350°F and grease a 9 × 5 inch loaf pan. Combine dry ingredients in a large bowl. Add egg replacement to the buttermilk mixture, then mix with the dry ingredients. Stir until blended, then mix in butter. Pour into prepared pan, bake for forty-five minutes or until a toothpick inserted comes out clean. Cool in pan or on wire rack.

Per serving (1/8 loaf):
Calories: 226
Fat (gm): 5
Carbohydrate (gm): 39
Protein (gm): 5
Fiber (gm): 2

95% Vegan Food Choices™:
2 grain

95% Vegan BUCs™: 3

Ambrosia Fruit Salad

Makes 16 servings

Ingredients:

You can really use whatever fruit you like in an ambrosia salad depending on how sweet or tart you want it to be, but this is what we like to use.

2 honeybell oranges, peeled and divided into segments
1 grapefruit, peeled and divided into segments
1 pomelo, peeled and divided into segments
1 can pineapple tidbits, drained
1 can light coconut milk
3 cups coconut flakes
1 recipe vegan marshmallows (recipe below)
½ cups chopped nuts of your choice (optional)
cherries (optional)

Combine all ingredients in a bowl, refrigerate 35–45 minutes before serving. For a sweeter salad, use canned Mandarin oranges or regular oranges peeled and divided into segments instead grapefruit and pomelo.

Per serving:
Calories: 109
Fat (gm): 6
Carbohydrate (gm): 14
Protein (gm): 1
Fiber (gm): 3

95% Vegan Food Choices™:
1 fruit
1 fat

95% Vegan BUCs™: 2

Vegan Marshmallows

Makes one 9 × 13 inch pan (24 servings)

Ingredients:
3 Tbsp. vegan gelatin (agar powder works well)
1 cup water
2 cup granulated sugar
¾ cup light corn syrup
¼ tsp. salt
1 Tbsp. vanilla

Combine all ingredients except water, vegan gelatin, and vanilla in a medium saucepan over high heat. Whisk ingredients together and bring up to 245°F. Remove from heat. Beat together the water and vegan gelatin, and combine with the syrup mixture. Beat together with electric mixer, and add vanilla. Beat the mixture for 15 minutes or so; it will begin to resemble marshmallow fluff. Dust a 9 × 13 inch pan with cornstarch or powdered sugar, pour the fluff into the pan. Refrigerate for 12 hours, remove from pan, and cut into marshmallow-size pieces.

Per serving:
Calories: 98
Fat (gm): 0
Carbohydrate (gm): 26
Protein (gm): 0
Fiber (gm): 0

95% Vegan Food Choices™:
1 ½ fruit

95% Vegan BUCs™:
2

Tamales

Makes 8 tamales

Ingredients:
1 cup TVP (texturized vegetable protein
1 cup Better Than Bouillon® No Beef Base (1 tsp. bouillon combined with 1 cup hot water)
1 medium onion, diced
2 Tbsp. soy sauce
1 tsp. ground cumin
2 cloves garlic, minced
8 flour tortillas
1 recipe Melty White Cheez from *The Ultimate Uncheese Cookbook* by Jo Stepaniak, reprinted in Appendix 2
guacamole and salsa to taste
2 Tbsp. olive oil

Combine TVP and broth in a large bowl, stir, and let sit for a few minutes. Add onions, soy sauce, garlic, and cumin. Spoon the mixture into the flour tortillas, roll, and place face down in a greased baking pan (or grill pan). Brush the tops of the tamales with the oil. You can choose to grill or bake the tamales in the pan. To bake, preheat oven to 350°F and cook for 10 minutes. To grill, place pan on grill over a low heat fire for 5–10 minutes—this will make the tamales smoky and delicious! Be careful not to burn the tamales on the grill, which is easy to do. Serve with guacamole and salsa to taste.

Per serving (1 tamale):
Calories: 260
Fat (gm): 9
Carbohydrate (gm): 34
Protein (gm): 12
Fiber (gm): 5

95% Vegan Food Choices™:
1 legume
1 grain
1 fat

95% Vegan BUCs™: 4

Tres Leches Cake

Makes 15 Servings

This cake comes out very soft; serve in a margarita glass and top with a cherry! For a more solid cake, reduce the amount of the mixed coconut cream, coconut milk, and soymilk mixture poured over the baked cake by half. This will make the cake less saturated and wet and would also reduce the amount of calories and fat in a serving.

Ingredients:
1-½ cup all-purpose flour
1 tsp. baking power
½ cup Earth Balance® vegan butter
1 cup sugar
5 Tbsp. egg replacer mixed with 15 Tbsp. water (you can measure
1 cup water and remove 1 Tbsp. to get 15 Tbsp.)
1 tsp. vanilla
½ tsp. salt
½ cup coconut cream
½ cup soy milk
1 can light coconut milk

Whipped topping:
1 can coconut cream
1 can regular fat coconut milk
1-½ cup powdered sugar
¼ cup cornstarch

Preheat over to 350°F and grease a 9 × 13 inch baking pan (The deeper the pan, the better, because a lot of liquid will be going in it!). Cream the Earth Balance® and sugar together. Add egg replacement mixture, salt, and vanilla, and beat well. Add the baking powder, and slowly add flour, mixing constantly until well-blended. Pour the batter into the pan, and bake for 30 minutes or until golden brown.

Pierce the cake all over with a fork; allow the cake to cool. Combine coconut cream, light coconut milk, and soymilk, and pour over the cake. Allow the cake to absorb all the milk.

Combine the whipped topping ingredients in a blender and whip on high. Pour over cake after it has absorbed the milks. Serve warm or chilled.

Per serving:
Calories: 428

Fat (gm): 18
Carbohydrate (gm): 65
Protein (gm): 3
Fiber (gm): 1

95% Vegan Food Choices™:
3 grain
2 fat

95% Vegan BUCs™:
7

Or

95% Vegan Food Choices™:
2 dessert

Banana Ice Cream Base

Makes 6 servings

Ingredients:
1 can regular coconut milk
2-½ large bananas, sliced and frozen
2 Tbsp. barley malt
2 cup vanilla soy milk
¼ cup brown sugar
¼ tsp. xanthan gum (optional for a more scoopable texture)

Combine all ingredients in blender, and blend on highest setting until smooth. Place in an ice cream maker—we use the ice cream maker bowl attachment for the KitchenAid®. Allow to churn for 15–20 minutes. Serve immediately or place in a freezer-safe container and freeze immediately.

Optional additions:
½ cup chopped nuts
¾ cup vegan chocolate chips
natural peanut butter

Per serving (without optional additives):
Calories: 176
Fat (gm): 5
Carbohydrate (gm): 57
Protein (gm): 3
Fiber (gm): 2

95% Vegan Food Choices™:
1.5 fruit
0.5 legume
0.5 fat

95% Vegan BUCs™: 3

Or

95% Vegan Food Choices: 1 dessert

Barbeque Ribs

Makes 10 large ribs

Ingredients:
2 cups vital wheat gluten
8 cups Better Than Bouillon® No Beef Base (8 tsp. bouillon combined with 8 cups hot water)
Tip: Remove 1-½ cup broth, and set the rest aside in a large pot.
1 tsp. Liquid Smoke®
2 Tbsp. soy sauce

½ bottle of your preferred barbeque sauce (we use the Jack Daniels® brand)
Cooking broth:
The set-aside 6 ½ cups broth
¼ cup brown sugar, packed
¼ cup soy sauce

Mix the cooking broth ingredients, and start in a large stockpot over high heat.

In a large bowl, combine vital wheat gluten, 1-½ cup broth, 2 Tbsp. soy sauce, and liquid smoke®. Mix thoroughly with a spoon, then knead by hand into a ball. Once the cooking broth comes to a boil, add the seitan dough, and boil the dough for 45 minutes. Remove the dough from the pot and let cool on a cutting board. Slice the seitan into quarter-inch-thick slices. Add the slices back to the broth and boil again for 15 minutes. Remove and let cool. Skewer the slices on bamboo skewers. Pour barbeque sauce into a large baking dish and lay the skewers in the pan; pour the rest of the barbeque sauce over the skewers. Refrigerate for 24 hours, take out of refrigerator, and let stand for 1 hour. Cook on a grill for 5 minutes on each side (or in a skillet if you prefer). Serve hot.

Per serving (1 rib):
Calories: 167
Fat (gm): 1
Carbohydrate (gm): 20
Protein (gm): 20
Fiber (gm): 1

95% Vegan Food Choices™:
1grain
0.5 legume

95% Vegan BUCs™: 2

"Sausage" Calzones

Makes 1 large calzone, 4 servings

Ingredients:
1 pre-prepared pizza dough or homemade dough
1 24 oz. jar tomato sauce
1 8 oz vegan mozzarella
1 Italian Tofurky® sausage, sliced thin
½ medium onion, diced
1 yellow squash, diced
Optional: Sprinkle nutritional yeast flakes inside or on top of the calzone for a cheesier taste and for increased protein, if desired.

Preheat oven to 350°F. Start skillet over medium heat. Add Tofurky®, onion, squash, and one-half jar of tomato sauce, and cook over medium heat for 10 minutes or until vegetables are tender. Roll dough to about ¼ inch thick. Spoon the contents of the skillet onto the dough, and sprinkle 4 oz of the vegan cheese into each calzone. Fold the dough over and tuck the ends to keep the filling from seeping out. Place on a greased cookie sheet with the tucked ends down and slice 1 to 3 slits in the top of the calzones to give the steam a place to escape. Bake for 20 minutes or until tops of calzones are golden brown. Serve while hot with remaining tomato sauce for dipping.

Per serving:
Calories: 688
Fat (gm): 27
Carbohydrate (gm): 87
Protein (gm): 22
Fiber (gm): 9

95% Vegan Food Choices™:

1 vegetable
1 legume
3.5 grain
3 fat

95% Vegan BUCs™:
10

Zeppoles

Makes 16 zeppoles

Ingredients:
1 cup all-purpose flour
2 tsp. baking powder
1 dash salt
½ Tbsp. sugar
2 Tbsp. flaxseed meal mixed with 6 Tbsp. water
1 cup Sweet Cheese (see page 365)
¼ tsp. vanilla
1 cup powdered sugar in a paper bag
canola oil, enough to fill a nonstick skillet 1 ½ to 2 inches

Start canola oil in a skillet over medium heat. Combine the rest of the ingredients except the powdered sugar, and mix well. Scoop by spoonfuls into hot oil. The zeppoles will start at the bottom of the skillet and rise to the top as they cook. They may turn over by themselves, but you may need to help them with a slotted spoon. Fry until both sides are golden brown. Drain and cool on a plate lined with paper towels. Place the cooled zeppoles into the bag of powdered sugar and toss, coating evenly with the sugar. Serve while warm.

Per serving (1 zeppole):
Calories: 142

Fat (gm): 8
Carbohydrate (gm): 17
Protein (gm): 2
Fiber (gm): 1

95% Vegan Food Choices™:
1 grain
1 fat

95% Vegan BUCs™:
3

Giant Soft Pretzels

Makes 12–13 pretzels

Ingredients:
Pretzel Dough:
6 cups all-purpose flour
1 Tbsp. active dry yeast
¾ cup nutritional yeast flakes
2-2/3 cups water
1 Tbsp. granulated garlic
1 tsp. salt
kosher salt

Baking Ingredients:
2 cups all-purpose flour on a clean, dry surface
¼ cup baking soda
6 cups water

Combine the pretzel dough ingredients in a large bowl, cover with a dish towel and leave to rise in a warm place for 40 minutes, allowing to double in size. Put the 6 cups water and ¼ cup baking soda in a large saucepan over high heat and bring to a boil. Turn dough out onto the heavily floured surface. Knead until the dough is workable. Divide into 12 to 13 equal pieces of dough; work each piece into a rope of dough, and form into pretzel shape. Preheat oven to 350°F. Dip each pretzel into the boiling water for 30 seconds, and place onto a greased cookie sheet. Repeat for each piece of dough. Sprinkle the uncooked pretzels with kosher salt to taste. Once completed, bake for 10 minutes or until golden brown.

Per serving (1 pretzel):
Calories: 317
Fat (gm): 1
Carbohydrate (gm): 65
Protein (gm): 10
Fiber (gm): 3

95% Vegan Food Choices™:
2.5 grain
0.5 legume

95% Vegan BUCs™:
5

Black Forest Oktoberfest Cake

Makes 12 servings

Ingredients:
Cake:
1 cup soy milk
1 Tbsp. white vinegar
1-¾ cup all-purpose flour
2 cup sugar
¾ cup cocoa powder
1 tsp. baking powder

2 tsp. baking soda
½ tsp. salt
2 Tbsp. ground flaxseed meal mixed with 6 Tbsp. water
½ cup canola oil
1 cup brewed coffee
1 Tbsp. vanilla

Cherry Filling:
    1 can cherry pie filling (or if you prefer a tart cherry flavor,
prepare your own by cooking down fresh or frozen cherries with
1 Tbsp. cornstarch and sugar to taste)
½ cup cherry liqueur

Whipped topping:
Either buy the pre-prepared soy whipped topping in a can or
blend until creamy:
12.3 oz package of soft silken tofu
½ cup powdered sugar and
2 Tbsp. lemon juice

Preheat oven to 350°F. Grease two 9-inch cake pans. Combine
cherry pie filling and cherry liqueur, and refrigerate the mixture
until icing the cake. Combine soy milk and vinegar, and set aside
to curdle. In a medium bowl, combine all dry ingredients (flour,
sugar, cocoa, baking powder, baking soda, salt). In a separate large
bowl, combine the wet ingredients for the cake (milk mixture,
flaxseed mixture, oil, coffee, vanilla). Gradually stir the flour mixture into the wet ingredients, mixing until combined (there will
be lumps). Pour into the cake pans, and cook for 25–30 minutes
or until a toothpick inserted comes out clean. Allow cakes to cool
in pan for 15 minutes before turning them out on a plate. Place
one cake face up on a plate and cover it with the cherry mixture.
Place the second cake on top. If your cake falls apart coming
out of the pan, you can put it in a large mixing bowl and mix

the cherry mixture in, forming a sticky dough. You can form the sticky dough into a cake, and it will be just as tasty!

Allow to completely cool before covering with a whipped soy topping. The cake will taste best after being set out for a day, so you may want to hold off on the whipped topping until the cake and cherry mixture have been combined 24 hours.

Per serving:
Calories: 332
Fat (gm): 9
Carbohydrate (gm): 61
Protein (gm): 4
Fiber (gm): 2

95% Vegan Food Choices™:
2 grain
1 fruit
1 fat

95% Vegan BUCs™:
5

Or

95% Vegan Food Choices™:
1.5 dessert

Vegan Liverwurst

Makes a 9 × 5 loaf, 10 servings

Ingredients:
9 × 5 loaf pan, greased

1 12.3 oz box silken tofu
4 oz red potato, peeled and sliced
½ medium onion, diced
¼ cup nutritional yeast flakes
¼ cup soy sauce
1-½ Tbsp. lemon juice
2 Tbsp. water
2 cloves garlic, minced
1 tsp. sugar
½ tsp. thyme
½ tsp. rosemary
½ tsp. marjoram
1/8 tsp. allspice

Preheat oven to 350°F. Combine all ingredients in a blender and process until very smooth. Pour into oiled loaf pan. Cover with foil and cook 90 minutes or until set. Uncover and cook for an additional 10–15 minutes.

Per serving:
Calories: 42
Fat (gm): 2
Carbohydrate (gm): 4
Protein (gm): 4
Fiber (gm): 0

95% Vegan Food Choices™:
0.5 legume

95% Vegan BUCs™:
1

Popcorn Balls

Makes 25 popcorn balls

Ingredients:
5 quarts plain popped popcorn in 2 large bowls
2 cups sugar
1 cup light corn syrup
½ cup Earth Balance® vegan butter
¼ cup water
salt to taste

Combine all ingredients except for popcorn in a medium saucepan. Whisk together over high heat. Using a candy thermometer, bring the caramel mixture up to 245°F. Pour the hot caramel over the popped popcorn, and allow it to cool for a few minutes. Then, using a large spoon, mix the caramel through the popcorn. Then, using your hands, form the caramel popcorn into 3–4 inch balls and enjoy! These stay good for several days.

Per serving (1 popcorn ball):
Calories: 157
Fat (gm): 4
Carbohydrate (gm): 31
Protein (gm): 1
Fiber (gm): 1

95% Vegan Food Choices™:
1 grain
1 fat

95% Vegan BUCs™:
3

Gooey Caramel Apples

Makes 8 servings

Ingredients:
8 small to medium organic apples, washed and dried (organic makes a difference in this recipe)
8 wooden popsicle sticks, stuck in the bottom of the apples
¼ cup vanilla soy yogurt
1 cup sugar
¾ cup dark corn syrup
1 Tbsp. Earth Balance® vegan butter
1 large bowl filled with ice water
one pan lined with wax paper

Combine yogurt, sugar, corn syrup, and Earth Balance in a saucepan, whisk over high heat. using a candy thermometer, bring the caramel to 245°F. Once the caramel reaches that temperature, remove the saucepan from heat and put it in the bowl of ice water. Allow caramel to cool and thicken for 4–5 minutes. Holding the stick, dip each apple into the caramel, cover evenly, allow excess to drip off, and place the apples top down in the lined pan. Put the pan with the apples in the refrigerator 20–30 minutes to help the caramel set before eating. The caramel will be gooey! You can set aside any unused caramel for future apples or as a caramel topping for another dessert. We encourage you to play around with the ingredients of your caramel mixture; you may find that you prefer a harder caramel consistency by using less yogurt. You can also roll a caramel-dipped apple in chopped nuts, sprinkles, or vegan chocolate shavings.

Per serving:
Calories: 281
Fat (gm): 2

Carbohydrate (gm): 71
Protein (gm): 0
Fiber (gm): 4

95% Vegan Food Choices™:
2 grain
1 fruit

95% Vegan BUCs™:
4

Vegan Thanksgiving Stuffing

Makes 10 servings

Ingredients:
1 tube Gimme Lean® vegan sausage
½ loaf white bread
3 Tbsp. flaxseed meal mixed with 9 Tbsp. water
½ yellow onion, diced

Preheat oven to 350°F. Dampen each slice of bread under running water. Then in a large bowl, combine all ingredients by hand and knead until well-mixed. Place in a greased casserole dish and cook uncovered for 30 minutes.

Per serving:
Calories: 114
Fat (gm): 2
Carbohydrate (gm): 19
Protein (gm): 7
Fiber (gm): 4

95% Vegan Food Choices™:
0.5 grain

0.5 legume

95% Vegan BUCs™:
2

Potato Latkes

Makes 6 latkes

Ingredients:
2 cups shredded potato squeezed in cheesecloth or paper towels
to remove moisture
1 Tbsp. grated onion (dried is fine)
3 Tbsp. flaxseed meal mixed with 9 Tbsp. water
2 Tbsp. all-purpose flour
1-½ tsp. salt
½ cup canola oil for frying
optional: apple sauce and vegan sour cream

   Mix all ingredients (except canola oil). Start a large nonstick
skillet over medium heat and add the canola oil. Once the oil is
hot, pour latke mixture in 6 equal lumps into skillet. Brown latke
on one side; flip, and brown on the other side. Serve while hot
with applesauce and vegan sour cream on the side, if desired.

Per serving (1 latke):
Calories: 230
Fat (gm): 20
Carbohydrate (gm): 13
Protein (gm): 2
Fiber (gm): 2

95% Vegan Food Choices™:
0.5 grain

3 fat

95% Vegan BUCs™:
4

Vegan Noodle Kugel

Makes 12 servings

Ingredients:
1 box lasagna, boiled, drained, and sliced width-wise into 1-inch slices
½ cup Earth Balance® vegan butter
3 recipes of sweet cheese, prepared (see recipe below)
1 cup sugar
6 Tbsp. egg replacer and 18 Tbsp. water mixed together
1 Tbsp. cinnamon
½ cup raisins

Preheat oven to 350°F. Combine prepared noodles and the rest of the ingredients. Pour into a greased baking dish (approximately 9 × 13 inches). Cover and bake until top is golden brown, about 25–30 minutes.

Per serving:
Calories: 310
Fat (gm): 9
Carbohydrate (gm): 51
Protein (gm): 9
Fiber (gm): 4

95% Vegan Food Choices™:
2 grain
0.5 legume

1 fat

95% Vegan BUCs™:
5

Blueberry Cheese Blintzes

Makes 6 Blintzes

Ingredients:
Crepe batter:
1 cup soy milk
¼ cup water
2 Tbsp. ground flaxseed mixed with 6 Tbsp. water (replacing 2 eggs)
1 cup all-purpose flour
pinch of salt
1 Tbsp. sugar
4 Tbsp. Earth Balance® vegan butter (3 Tbsp. in crepe batter and 1 Tbsp. for sautéing crepes)
sweet cheese, prepared (see recipe below)
blueberry filling (see recipe below)

Combine crepe batter ingredients in blender; blend until extremely smooth (Chunks are okay for pancakes, not crepes!). Put batter in refrigerator for at least 1 hour. Preheat oven to 350°F. Put a nonstick skillet over medium heat, and add remaining tablespoon of Earth Balance to skillet. Pour batter into skillet in 1/3 cup amounts. The crepes will start to bubble and dry around the edges. Once the crepes have bubbles all over and the edges are thoroughly dry (but not burned), flip them with a spatula. Allow to cook for a minute, and then remove to a plate. Lay crepes flat; fill with cheese and/or blueberry filling as desired. Roll up crepes, and add them to a greased pan. Put the pan in the oven for 5–10 minutes; serve while hot.

Per serving (1 crepe with 1 serving each sweet cheese and blueberry filling):
Calories: 352
Fat (gm): 13
Carbohydrate (gm): 53
Protein (gm): 7
Fiber (gm): 3

95% Vegan Food Choices™:
1 grain
1 legume
1 fruit
1.5 fat

95% Vegan BUCs™:
6

Sweet Cheese

Makes 6 servings

Ingredients:
One 12.3 oz box soft silken tofu
2 Tbsp. lemon juice
½ cup powered sugar (more or less to taste)

Combine ingredients in a blender; blend until smooth.

Per serving:
Calories: 72

Fat (gm): 2
Carbohydrate (gm): 12
Protein (gm): 4
Fiber (gm): 0

95% Vegan Food Choices™:
0.5 legume

95% Vegan BUCs™:
1

Blueberry Filling

Makes 10 servings

Ingredients:
2 Tbsp. Earth Balance® vegan butter
10 oz frozen blueberries
¾ cup sugar
1 Tbsp. cornstarch
2 Tbsp. lemon juice

Combine ingredients in a saucepan. Bring to a boil for 10–15 minutes, cool, and set aside. It will thicken as it cools.

Per serving:
Calories: 100
Fat (gm): 2
Carbohydrate (gm): 19
Protein (gm): 0
Fiber (gm): 1

95% Vegan Food Choices™:
2 fruit

95% Vegan BUCs™:
2

Bread Machine Vegan Challah

Makes 2-pound loaf (16 servings)

(Thanks to Marcy Saucedo for sharing her recipe!)

Ingredients:
1 cup soy milk
3 Tbsp. flaxseed meal and 9 Tbsp. water (to replace 3 eggs)
4 Tbsp. Earth Balance® vegan butter
4 cups bread flour
1/3 cup sugar
1-2/3 tsp. salt
2 tsp. active dry yeast
¼ cup olive or flaxseed oil

Add all ingredients to bread machine set on a "dough" setting. When dough is finished, remove dough, set in greased bowl, cover, and keep in warm place. Allow dough to double in size. Preheat oven to 375°F. When doubled, place on floured board and knead a few times. Separate into 3 equal pieces and roll into long cords. Braid the 3 cords. Tuck in ends. Brush top with oil. Bake 20–25 minutes or until crust is dark golden brown. Brush again with oil. Yields 1 very large loaf. You can divide dough into 6 cords and have 2 small loaves.

Per serving:
Calories: 209
Fat (gm): 8
Carbohydrate (gm): 31
Protein (gm): 5
Fiber (gm): 1

95% Vegan Food Choices™:
1.5 grain
1 fat

95% Vegan BUCs™:
3

African-Style Peanut Soup

Makes 6 Servings

Ingredients:
4 cups Better Than Bouillon® No Chicken Base (4 tsp. bouillon combined with 4 cups hot water)
1 medium onion, diced
1 large sweet potato, cubed
1 sweet pepper, diced
1 cup plain peanut butter
1 tsp. salt (more or less to taste)
pepper to taste

Combine all ingredients in a Crock-Pot®, and cook on low heat for 5–8 hours. Serve while hot.

Per serving:
Calories: 306
Fat (gm): 22
Carbohydrate (gm): 21
Protein (gm): 12
Fiber (gm):5

95% Vegan Food Choices™:
0.5 grain
1 legume

3 fat

95% Vegan BUCs™:
5

Cornbread

Makes one 8 × 5 inch loaf (8–10 servings)

Ingredients:
1 cup self-rising flour
1 cup yellow cornmeal
1 tsp. salt
¼ cup sugar
¼ cup canola oil
1 cup plain soy milk
2 Tbsp. ground flaxseed mixed with 6 Tbsp. water

Preheat oven to 400°F. Combine all ingredients in a large bowl, and mix well. Pour batter into greased loaf pan or muffin tins if you prefer. Cook for 25–30 minutes or until set and golden brown on top.

Per serving (1/10 loaf):
Calories: 186
Fat (gm): 7
Carbohydrate (gm): 29
Protein (gm): 3
Fiber (gm): 2

95% Vegan Food Choices™:
1 grain
1 fat

95% Vegan BUCs™:

3

Jiaozi-Chinese Dumplings

Makes 25 Servings

Ingredients:
Dumpling Dough:
3 cups all-purpose dough
¼ tsp. salt
1-¼ cup water (you may not use all of it)

Dumpling filling:
1 cup TVP
1 cup Better Than Bouillon® No Chicken Base (1 tsp. bouillon combined with 1 cup hot water)
1 Tbsp. soy sauce
¼ tsp. white pepper
3 Tbsp. flaxseed oil
½ cup green onion, diced
1 yellow onion, diced
1 large slice ginger, minced
1 clove garlic, minced

These are just suggested filling ingredients; you can choose a wide variety of filling items. Cabbage and bamboo shoots are great for an authentic Chinese dumpling, but you can also use peppers or other vegetables.

Preparing the dough:
Combine the flour and salt. Slowly mix in the water, and stir until it forms a ball of dough; you may not need all of the water. Set aside.

Preparing the filling:

Combine the TVP and broth, stir, and set aside. Start a skillet over medium heat, and add flax oil. When hot, add the onions, and sauté. When the onions are soft, add the TVP and the rest of the dumpling filling to the skillet. Mix and heat thoroughly, set aside, and allow to cool.

Making the dumplings:
Start boiling 10 cups water in a large stockpot. Divide the dumpling dough into 25–30 equal pieces. Roll the dough flat and thin, spoon 1-½ to 2 Tbsp. of the filling into the flat dumpling. Fold the dough over, and roll and pinch shut the edges, sealing them well. When the pot of water is boiling, add the dumplings, gently using a wooden spoon to separate any dumplings stuck together. Bring back to a boil. Add 1 cup cold water into the pot. Bring it to a boil again. Repeat this process once more, and your dumplings are done and ready to eat!

Per serving:
Calories: 85
Fat (gm): 2
Carbohydrate (gm): 13
Protein (gm): 4
Fiber (gm): 1

95% Vegan Food Choices™:
0.5 grain
0.5 legume

95% Vegan BUCs™:
2

Buffalo Chick'n Patties

Makes 8 patties

Ingredients:
Cutlets:
1-¼ cups vital wheat gluten
½ cup Better Than Bouillon® No Chicken Base (½ tsp. bouillon combined with ½ cup hot water)
¼ cup soy sauce
1 Tbsp. flaxseed oil
1 Tbsp. granulated garlic

Cooking broth:
6 cups Better Than Bouillon® No Chicken Base (6 tsp. bouillon combined with 6 cup hot water)
¼ cup soy sauce

Buffalo preparation:
¼ cup flour for flouring chick'n
¼ cup canola oil for frying
2 cup all-purpose flour
1 bottle Frank's RedHot® Original sauce

Start cooking broth over high heat, and bring to the boil. In the meantime, combine the dry ingredients of the cutlets and blend. Then add the broth, soy sauce, and oil to the dry ingredients, and stir with a spoon until combine. Then knead by hand until you have a smooth ball of dough. Place the dough ball into the boiling cooking broth and reduce to a simmer, simmering for 1 hour. Remove the cooked chick'n and place on a plate to cool. Start ¼ cup of the canola oil in a large skillet on medium-high heat. Slice the chick'n into 6 equal pieces. Toss the slices in the remaining canola oil to coat. Place the 2 cups all-purpose flour in a bowl, and toss the oiled slices in the flour, coating evenly. Then place the floured slices into the skillet, lightly cooking on both sides, then evenly pour Frank's RedHot® Original sauce over slices, covering completely. Cook on both sides again. Remove from skillet, and serve on a bun or sliced into chick'n fingers.

Plain Fried Chick'n Variation:
    Simply don't add the Frank's RedHot Original sauce, and presto, plain chick'n patties or fingers!

Per serving (1 buffalo chick'n patty):
Calories: 328
Fat (gm): 14
Carbohydrate (gm): 7
Protein (gm): 16
Fiber (gm): 1

95% Vegan Food Choices™:
2 grain
2 fat

95% Vegan BUCs™:
5

Mardi Gras King Cake [Rosca de Reyes]

Makes 2 large cakes

Ingredients:
Pastry:
1 cup soy milk
¼ cup Earth Balance® vegan butter

4 tsp. active dry yeast
2/3 cup warm water
½ cup white sugar
2 Tbsp. ground flaxseed mixed with 6 Tbsp. water
1 ½ tsp. salt
½ tsp. nutmeg
5-½ cup all-purpose flour

Filling:
1 cup packed brown sugar
1 Tbsp. ground cinnamon
2/3 cup chopped pecans (or 1 cup pecan halves)
½ cup all-purpose flour
½ cup raisins
½ cup melted butter

Frosting:
1 cup powdered sugar
1 Tbsp. water
colored sugars (purple, yellow, and green)

Preparing the pastry:
Warm soymilk in microwave or on stove top, add butter, mix together, and set aside to cool. In a large bowl, combine yeast and warm water, and set aside for 5–10 minutes. Add the milk and butter mixture to the yeast, whisk in egg mixture. Whisk in white sugar, salt, and nutmeg. Slowly add flour to the wet ingredients until completely combined. Turn out on a floured surface, and knead until elastic. Add oil to the mixing bowl and oil the sides of the bowl. Return dough ball to the bowl, and turn it over a few times to coat the dough ball in oil. Set aside at room temperature or in a warm oven and allow to rise for an hour or until the dough has doubled in size. Punch down the dough and cut in half.

Preparing the filling:

Combine the filling ingredients in a food processor, and blend until uniform.

Making the cakes:

Roll out the dough half to a large rectangle; add a line of filling down the middle lengthwise. Roll the cake up like a jelly roll, form the roll into a ring, and connect the ends. Lay out on a cookie sheet lined with wax paper. Slit the top of the cake ring every 3 inches. Repeat the process with the other half of the pastry dough. Leave the cakes at room temperature or in a warm oven; the cakes will double in size. Preheat the oven to 375°F, bake the cakes for 30 minutes, and let cool slightly. Frost the cakes while they are warm, and sprinkle the colored sugars while the icing is still wet.

Per serving (1/12 slice of one cake):
Calories: 282
Fat (gm): 8
Carbohydrate (gm): 49
Protein (gm): 4
Fiber (gm): 1

95% Vegan Food Choices™:
2 grain
1 fat

95% Vegan BUCs™:
4

Crock-Pot® Jambalaya

8 Servings

Ingredients:
2 Italian Tofurky® sausages cut into 1/8 inch pieces
1 can red kidney beans
2 Tbsp. canola oil
2 Tbsp. Cajun seasoning
1 onion, diced
1 10 oz bag frozen peppers
2 stalks celery, diced
4 cloves garlic, minced
1-16 oz can diced tomatoes
1 tsp. salt
1 tsp. hot sauce
2 tsp. vegan Worcestershire sauce
1 tsp. file sauce (optional)
1 ¼ cup uncooked long grain rice (white or brown)
8 cups Better Than Bouillon® No Chicken Base (8 tsp. bouillon combined with 8 cups hot water)

Combine all ingredients in a large crockpot, turn on low heat setting, and let cook for 5–8 hours. Serve while hot.

Per serving:
Calories: 296
Fat (gm): 7
Carbohydrate (gm): 45
Protein (gm): 13
Fiber (gm): 8

95% Vegan Food Choices™:
1 grain

1 legume
1 vegetables
1 fat

95% Vegan BUCs™:
4

Beignets

Makes 20 large beignets

Ingredients:
1 1/8 tsp. active dry yeast
¾ cup warm (not hot) water
¼ cup sugar
½ tsp. salt
1 Tbsp. flaxseed meal mixed with 3 Tbsp. water
¼ cup coconut cream
¼ cup soy milk
2 Tbsp. shortening
3-½ cups all-purpose flour

For cooking:
Oil (enough to fill nonstick skillet 1 ½ to 2 inches)
¼ cup powdered sugar for sprinkling

In a large bowl, combine yeast and warm water, blend, and let sit for 5 minutes. Add sugar, salt, coconut cream, soymilk, flaxseed mixture, and shortening, and blend well. Slowly add in the flour and mix until smooth. Let the mixture sit at room temperature to rise, allowing it to double in size. Put the dough in a refrigerator for at least 24 hours. After 24 hours, remove dough from refrigerator. Add oil to skillet over medium heat. Using your hands, make golf ball–sized dough balls, and place them in the oil. The dough should initially sink in the oil but will pop up to the top as they cook. Allow them to brown on one side, and flip, allowing them to brown on the other side. The beignets may flip themselves, but a slotted spoon may be needed to help. Remove from oil with the slotted spoon and pile the beignets on a plate. Allow them to cool a bit before sprinkling with powered sugar, and enjoy!

Per serving (1 beignet):
Calories: 216
Fat (gm): 13
Carbohydrate (gm): 23
Protein (gm): 3
Fiber (gm): 1

95% Vegan Food Choices™:
1 grain
2 fat

95% Vegan BUCs™:
4

Chocolate-Covered Strawberries

Makes 30 Servings

Ingredients:
2 pints fresh strawberries, washed and dried
1 bag vegan chocolate chips *or*
3 bars vegan dark chocolate

Many chocolates are already vegan; you just need to check the label for any milk, casein, or whey products.

Start a pot of hot water over medium-high heat. Lay out a sheet of waxed paper. Add a double boiler to the pot and place chocolate in the double boiler. [Double boilers help to melt chocolate without burning it.] Once the chocolate is melted, dip the strawberries in the chocolate holding the strawberries by their green tops. Place the dipped strawberries on the wax paper, and allow the chocolate to dry. Surprise your special someone with this delicious treat!

Per serving:
Calories: 61
Fat (gm): 3
Carbohydrate (gm): 9
Protein (gm): 1
Fiber (gm): 1

95% Vegan Food Choices™:
1 fruit

95% Vegan BUCs™:
1

APPENDIX 6

. . . .

95% VEGAN FOOD CHOICE PLAN PORTIONS

Legumes (approximately 110 calories, 8gm protein, 2gm fat, 15gm carbohy-drate, 6gm fiber, 1.5BUCs per serving)	Serving Size
Soy Milk, regular fat	1 cup
Soy Milk, light	1-1/2 cup
Beans (red, black, white)	1/2 of 15oz can or 3-1/2 oz dried, cooked
Chick Peas	1/2 cup cooked
Tofu	4 oz
Split Peas	1/2 cup cooked
Soy Tempeh	2 oz
Soy Yogurt	4 oz
Soy Beans (Edamame in Shell)	4 oz
Soy Beans, shelled	3 oz
Green Peas	5 oz
TVP (texturized vegetable protein)	1/3 cup dry
Nutritional Yeast Flakes	1/2 cup cooked
Legume Flours (soy, garbanzo, etc.)	1/4 cup

Grains (approximately 110 calories, 4gm protein, 1.5gm fat, 20gm carbohydrate, 2gm fiber, 1.5BUCs per serving)	Serving Size
Corn	1 cup
Potato, white	4 oz
Potato, sweet	1-1/2 oz
Bread, whole grain	1-1/2 oz
Rice, cooked	1/2 cup
Pasta, cooked	3 oz
Noodles, cooked	3 oz
Grain Flours (wheat, rye, oat, etc.)	1/4 cup
Winter Squash (acorn, butternut, etc.)	10 oz cooked
Pretzels	1 oz
Popcorn, popped	4 cups

Vegetables (approximately 25calories, 2gm protein, 0gm fat, 4gm carbohydrate, 2gm fiber, 0.25BUCs per serving)	1 cup raw or 1/2 cup cooked except where noted
Broccoli	
Spinach	
Carrots	
Cabbage	
Cauliflower	
Tomatoes	
Summer Squash (yellow, zucchini)	
Cucumber, 1 medium	

Fruits (approximately 60 calories, 0 gm protein, 0gm fat, 15gm carbohydrate, 3gm fiber, 1BUC per serving)	Serving Size
Apples	4 oz, no core
Oranges	4 oz
Tangerines	2 oz
Berries (strawberries, blackberries, blueberries, etc.)	4 oz
Dried Fruit	3/4 oz
Watermelon	8 oz
Peaches/Nectarines	6 oz
Cherries	3 oz
Grapes	3 oz
Banana	2-1/2 oz

Fats (approximately 50 calories, 0gm protein, 6gm fat, 0gm carbohydrate, 0gm fiber per serving)	Serving Size
Nuts	1/4 oz
Avocado	1 oz
Olives	1/2 Tbsp
Vegan Butter	1/2 Tbsp
Oils	1/2 Tbsp
Flax Seed	1/2 Tbsp

Desserts (approximately 200 calories, 2gm protein, 10gm fat, 26gm carbohydrate, 1gm fiber, 3 BUCs per serving)
Do not exceed calorie amount

Condiments (approximately 50 calories, macronutrient content varies, 1BUC per serving)	Serving Size
Catsup	4 Tbsp
Sugar	1 Tbsp
Honey	2-1/2 tsp

Misc.	Choices per Serving	BUCs per serving
Potato Chips, 1oz.	1 grain, 1 fat	3
Granola Bar, 1	1 grain, 1 fat	3
Biscuit, 1 medium (2-1/2 inches wide)	1 grain, 1/2 fat	2

APPENDIX 7

· ·

YOUR TURN: 7 DAY MEAL PLAN

7 Day Meal Plan for 95% Vegan Calorie Counting™   Calories per day:_____

Day:	Breakfast	Calories	Lunch	Calories	Dinner	Calories	Snack	Calories	Snack	Calories	Snack	Calories
1												
2												
3												
4												
5												
6												
7												

7 Day Meal Plan for the 95% Vegan Food Choice Plan™   Choices per Day

Legume:_____   Grain:_____   Fruit:_____   Vegetable:_____   Fat:_____

Dessert:_____   Condiment:_____

Day:	Breakfast	Choices	Lunch	Choices	Dinner	Choices	Snack	Choices	Snack	Choices	Snack	Choices
1												
2												
3												
4												
5												
6												
7												

7 Day Meal Plan for the 95% Vegan BUC Plan™   BUCs per day:_____

Day	Breakfast	BUCs	Lunch	BUCs	Dinner	BUCs	Snack	BUCs	Snack	BUCs	Snack	BUCs	Total BUCS
1													
2													
3													
4													
5													
6													
7													

APPENDIX 8

· ·

YOUR DIABETES SNAPSHOT

Date:		Day of Week:				
Fasting (before breakfast)	2 hrs after breakfast	Before lunch	2 hrs after lunch	Before supper	2 hrs after supper	Bedtime

Date:		Day of Week:				
Fasting (before breakfast)	2 hrs after breakfast	Before lunch	2 hrs after lunch	Before supper	2 hrs after supper	Bedtime

Date:		Day of Week:				
Fasting (before breakfast)	2 hrs after breakfast	Before lunch	2 hrs after lunch	Before supper	2 hrs after supper	Bedtime

Date:		Day of Week:				
Fasting (before breakfast)	2 hrs after breakfast	Before lunch	2 hrs after lunch	Before supper	2 hrs after supper	Bedtime

Date:		Day of Week:					
Fasting (before breakfast)	2 hrs after breakfast	Before lunch	2 hrs after lunch	Before supper	2 hrs after supper	Bedtime	

Date:		Day of Week:					
Fasting (before breakfast)	2 hrs after breakfast	Before lunch	2 hrs after lunch	Before supper	2 hrs after supper	Bedtime	

Date:		Day of Week:					
Fasting (before breakfast)	2 hrs after breakfast	Before lunch	2 hrs after lunch	Before supper	2 hrs after supper	Bedtime	

REFERENCES

Introduction

1. T. Colin Campbell and Thomas M. Campbell, *The China Study* (2006).

2. Caldwell B. Esselstyn Jr., *Prevent and Reverse Heart Disease* (2007).

3. *Forks Over Knives* (2011) available on DVD.

4. "The Diabetes Prevention Program Research Group," *New England Journal of Medicine* 346, no. 6 (2002): 393–403.

5. The American Diabetes Association (2009)

Part I:
A Marriage of Science, Society and Your Realities

My Story

1. Hope R. Ferdowsian et al., "A Multicomponent Intervention Reduces Body Weight and Cardiovascular Risk

at a GEICO Corporate Site," *American Journal of Health Promotion* 24, no. 6 (July/August 2010): 384–387.

2. Brenda Davis and Vesanto Melina, *Becoming Vegan* (2000).

3. Jo Stepaniak, *The Ultimate Uncheese Cookbook* (2003).

4. T. Colin Campbell and Thomas M. Campbell, *The China Study* (2006).

Why Vegan?

1. Winston J. Craig, "Health Effects of Vegan Diets," *American Journal of Clinical Nutrition* 89 (2009): 1627S-33S.

2. T. Colin Campbell and Thomas M. Campbell, *The China Study* (2006).

3. Caldwell B. Esselstyn Jr., *Prevent and Reverse Heart Disease* (2007).

4. Timothy J. Key et al., "Diet Nutrition and the Prevention of Cancer," *Public Health Nutrition* 7(1A) (2004): 187–200.

5. International Agency for Research on Cancer, "Cancer: Causes, Occurrence and Control," *IARC Scientific Publications* no. 100 (1990), Lyon: IARC.

6. Riccardo Baschetti, "Diabetes Epidemic in Newly Westernized Populations: Is it Due to Thrift Genes or to Genetically Unknown Foods?" *Journal of the Royal Society of Medicine* 91 (December 1998): 622–625.

7. "Position of the American Dietetic Association and Dietitians of Canada: Vegetarian Diets," *Journal of The*

American Dietetic Association 103, no. 6 (June 2003): 748–765.

Why 95% Vegan?

1. Caldwell B. Esselstyn Jr., *Prevent and Reverse Heart Disease* (2007).

2. The Harris Benedict Equation, available at http://www.bmi-calculator.net/bmr-calculator/bmr-formula.php.

3. Food values in this chapter were obtained from www.MyNetDiary.com.

4. http://www.atkinsexposed.org/atkins/95/margo_a._denke,_m.d..htm.

5. http://xnet.kp.org/permanentejournal/sum03/registry.html.

6. www.calorieking.com. The reference book is also available from many book stores.

The Importance of Learning How to Fish

1. www.brookes.ac.uk/services/ocsd. June 27, 2002

Creating a Ripple Effect, Generation to Generation

1. National Center for Health Statistics Health E-Stats, "Prevalence of Overweight, Obesity, and Extreme Obesity Among Adults: United States, Trends 1976–80 through 2005–2006" (2008).

2. Ogden CL et al., "Prevalence of Obesity in the United States, 2009–2010," NCHS data brief, no. 82 (2012), Hyattsville MD: National Center for Health Statistics, 2012.

3. http://win.niddk.nih.gov/publications/PDFs/stat904z.pdf

4. http://www.npr.org/blogs/thesalt/2012/06/27/1555 27365/visualizing-a-nation-of-meat-eaters

5. Joel Kimmons et al., "Fruit and Vegetable Intake Among Adolescents and Adults in the United States: Percentage Meeting Individualized Recommendations," *The Medscape Journal of Medicine* 11 (1) (2009): 26. Available at http://www.ncbi.nlm.nih.gov/pmc/articles/PMC2654704/

Part II:
First Things First

Home-Based Assessments for Nutritional Health Status

1. Eric J. Jacobs, et.al., "Waist Circumference and All-Cause Mortality in a Large U.S. Cohort," *Arch Intern Med 2010*, 170 (15) (2010): 1293–1301.

2. Ian Janssen, Peter Katzmarzyk, and Robert Ross, "Body Mass Index, Waist Circumference, and Health Risk, Evidence in Support of Current National Insitutes of Health Guidelines," *Arch Intern Med* 162 (2002): 2074–2079.

3. Dympa Gallagher et al., "Healthy Percentage Body Fat Ranges: An Approach for Developing Guidelines Based on Body Mass Index," *Am. J. Clin. Nutr 2000* vol. 72 (2000): 694–701.

4. Andres S. Levey et.al., "National Kidney Foundation Practice Guidelines for Chronic Kidney Disease: Evaluation, Classification and Stratification," *Ann Intern Med* 139 (2003): 137–147. Available at http://www.kidney.org/professionals/kdoqi/pdf/Med2003CKDguideline.pdf

5. http://www.nlm.nih.gov/medlineplus/ency/article/002222.htm

6. Michael F. Holick and Tai C. Chen, "Vitamin D Deficiency: A Worldwide Problem with Health Consequences, *Am J Clin Nutrition* 87 (suppl) (2008):1080S-6S.

7. Thomas J. Wang et.al., "Vitamin D Deficiency and Risk of Cardiovascular Disease," *Circulation* 117 (2008): 503–511.

8. "NCEP Report: Implications of Recent Clinical Trials for the National Cholesterol Education Program Adult Treatment Panel III Guidelines." Available at http://www.nhlbi.nih.gov/guidelines/cholesterol/atp3upd04.pdf

9. Paul S. Jellinger et.al., "American Association of Clinical Endocrinologists' Guidelines for Management of Dyslipidemia and Prevention of Atherosclerosis," *Endocrine Practice* 18 (Suppl 1) (March/April 2012).

10. Sabine Kahl and Michael Roden, "An Update on the Pathogenesis of Type 2 Diabetes Mellitus," *Hamdan Medical Journal 2012* 5 (2012): 99–122.

11. Terry W. Du Clos, "Function of C-Reactive Protein," *Annals of Medicine* 32, no. 4 (2000): 274–278.

12. Paul M. Ridker, Robert J. Glynn, and Charles H. Hennekens, "C-Reactive Protein Adds to the Predictive Value of Total and HDL Cholesterol in Determining Risk of First Myocardial Infarction," *Circulation* 97 (1998): 2007–2011.

13. Paul M. Ridker et al., "Prospective Study of C-Reactive Protein and the Risk of Future Cardiovascular Events Among Apparently Healthy Women," *Circulation* 98 (1998): 731–733.

14. Katherine Esposito et al., "Effect of a Mediterranean-Style Diet on Endothelial Dysfunction and Markers of Vascular Inflammation in the Metabolic Syndrome." *JAMA* 292, no. 12 (Sept 22/29, 2004): 1440–1446.

15. David J.A. Jenkins, et al., "Effects of a Dietary Portfolio of Cholesterol-Lowering Foods vs Lovastatin on Serum Lipids and C-Reactive Protein," *JAMA* 290, no. 4 (July 23/30): 502–510.

16. Earl S. Ford, "Does Exercise Reduce Inflammation? Physical Activity and C-Reactive Protein Among U.S. Adults" (2002).

17. Steven E. Nissen et al., "Statin Therapy, LDL Cholesterol, C-Reactive Protein, and Coronary Artery Disease," *New England Journal of Medicine 2005* 352 (2005): 29–38.

18. P. M. Ridker et al., "Rosuvastatin to Prevent Vascular Events in Men and Women with Elevated C-Reactive Protein," *New England Journal of Medicine 2008* 359 (2008): 2195–2207.

19. Richard M. Green and Steven Flamm, "AGA Technical Review on the Evaluation of Liver Chemistry Tests," *Gastroenterology* 123, 4 (October 2002):1367–1384.

The Macronutrients: Carbohydrate, Fat, and Protein

1. Nancy F. Sheard et al., "Dietary Carbohydrate (Amount and Type) in the Prevention and Management of Diabetes," *Diabetes Care* 27, no. 9 (September 2004) 2266–2271.

2. Dena M. Bravata et al., "Efficacy and Safety of Low-Carbohydrate Diets—A Systematic Review," *JAMA* 289, no. 14 (April 9, 2003): 1837–1850.

3. J. Salmeron et al., "Dietary Fiber, Glycemic Load, and Risk of Non-Insulin-Dependent Diabetes Mellitus in Women," *JAMA* 277 (1997): 472–477.

4. David S. Ludwig, "The Glycemic Index—Physiological Mechanisms Relating to Obesity, Diabetes and Cardiovascular Disease," *JAMA* 287, no. 18 (2002): 2414–2423.

5. Elissa S. Epel et al., "Cell Aging in Relation to Stress Arousal and Cardiovascular Disease Risk Factors," *Psychoneuroendocrinology* 31 (2006): 277–287.

6. Paul H. Black, "The Inflammatory Response Is an Integral Part of the Stress Response: Implications for Atherosclerosis, Insulin Resistance, Type II Diabetes and Metabolic Syndrome X." *Brain, Behavior, and Immunity* 17 (2002): 350–364.

7. Gong Yang et al., "Population-Based, Case Control Study of Blood C-Peptide Level and Breast Cancer Risk," *Cancer, Epidemiology, Biomarkers and Prevention* 10 (2001): 1207–1211.

8. U. Smith, E. A. M. Gale, "Does Diabetes Therapy Influence the Risk of Cancer?" *Diabetologia* 52 (2009): 1699–1708.

9. Dariush Mozaffarian et al., "Trans Fatty Acids and Cardiovascular Disease," *New England Journal of Medicine* 354, 15 (2006): 1601–6013.

10. Joseph R. Hibbeln et al., "Healthy Intakes of n-3 and n-6 Fatty Acids: Estimations Considering Worldwide Diversity," *Am J Clin Nutr 2006* 83 (suppl) (2006): 1483S-93S.William S. Harris et al. (2009).

11. "Omega-6 Fatty Acids and Risk for Cardiovascular Disease: A Science Advisory from the American Heart Association Nutritional Subcommittee for the Council on Nutrition, Physical Activity, and Metabolism; Council on Cardiovascular Nursing; and Council on Epidemiology and Prevention," *Circulation 2009* 119: 902–907.

12. Wayne W. Campbell et al., "Dietary Protein Requirements of Younger and Older Adults," *Am. J. Clin. Nutr. 2008* 88 (2008): 1322–1329.

13. Mohammad A. Humayun et al., "Reevaluation of the Protein Requirement in Young Men with the Indicator Amino Acid Oxidation Technique," *Am. J. Clin. Nutr.* 86 (2007): 995–1002.

14. Douglas Paddon-Jones et al., "Role of Dietary Protein in the Sarcopenia of Aging," *Am. J. Clin. Nutr.* 87 (suppl), pp. 1562S-1566S.

15. Jane E. Kerstetter, et.al. "Dietary Protein Affects Intestinal Calcium Absorption," *Am. J. Clin. Nutr.* 68 (1998): 859–865.

16. Marian T. Hannan et al., "Effect of Dietary Protein on Bone Loss in Elderly Men and Women: The Framingham Osteoporosis Study," *Journal of Bone and Mineral Research* 15, no. 12 (2000): 2504–2512.

17. William M. Rand et al., "Meta-Analysis of Nitrogen Balance Studies for Estimating Protein Requirements in Healthy Adults," *Am. J. Clin. Nutr.* 77 (2003): 109–127.

18. Vernon R. Young and Peter L. Pellet, "Plant Proteins in Relation to Human Protein and Amino Acid Nutrition," *Am. J. Clin. Nutr.* 59 (Suppl) (1994): 1203S-1212S.

19. Anna H. Wu et al., "Adolescent and Adult Soy Intake and Risk of Breast Cancer in Asian-Americans," *Carcinogenesis* 23, no. 9 (2002): 1491–1496.

20. Xiao Ou Shu et al., "Soyfood Intake During Adolescence and Subsequent Risk of Breast Cancer Among Chinese Women," *Cancer, Epidemiology, Biomarkers Prevention* 10 (May 2001): 483–488.

21. Leena Hilakivi-Clarke et al., "Is Soy Consumption Good or Bad for the Breast?" *The Journal of Nutrition, Supplement: Soy Summit—Exploration of the Nutrition and Health Effects of Whole Soy* 140 (2010): 2326S–2334S, 2010.

22. M. K. Kim et al., "Dietary Intake of Soy Protein and Tofu in Association with Breast Cancer Risk Based on a Case-Control Study," *Nutr. Cancer* 60 (5) (2008): 568–76.

23. Bruce J. Trock et al., "Meta-Analysis of Soy Intake and Breast Cancer Risk," *Journal of the National Cancer Institute* 98, no. 7 (April 6, 2006).

24. S. J. Nechuta et al., "Soy Food Intake After Diagnosis of Breast Cancer and Survival: An In-Depth Analysis of Combined Evidence from Cohort Studies of U.S. and Chinese Women," *Am. J. Clin. Nutr.* 96 (1) (July 2012): 123–32.

25. Dennis Paustenbach et al., "Human Health Risk and Exposure Assessment of Chromium (VI) in Tap Water," *Journal of Toxicology and Environmental Health, Part A: Current Issues* 66, 17 (2003).

26. M. J. Hooth, "Technical Report on Toxicology and Carcinogenesis Studies of Sodium Dichromate Dihydrate (CAS No. 7789-12-0) in F344/N Rats and B6C3F1 Mice (Drinking Water Studies)," (DIANE Publishing, 2009).

27. Karen A. Kidd et al., "Collapse of a Fish Population After Exposure to a Synthetic Estrogen," *PNAS (Proceedings of the National Academy of Sciences of the United States of America* 104, no. 21 (May 22, 2007).

28. Joanne L. Slavin, "Dietary Fiber and Body Weight," *Nutrition* 21, 3 (March 2005): 411–418.

29. James W. Anderson et al., "Carbohydrate and Fiber Recommendations for Individuals with Diabetes: A Quantitative Assessment and Meta-Analysis of the Evidence," *J Am Coll Nutr* 23, no. 1 (February 2004): 5–17.

30. Yikyung Park et al., "Dietary Fiber Intake and Risk of Colorectal Cancer, A Pooled Analysis of Prospective Cohort Studies," *JAMA* 29 (22) (2005): 2849–2857.

31. S. P. Whelton et al., "Effect of Dietary Fiber Intake on Blood Pressure: A Meta-Analysis of Randomized, Controlled Clinical Trials," *J Hypertens* 23 (2005): 475–481.

32. J. L. Slavin, "Position of the American Dietetic Association: Health Implications of Dietary Fiber," *Journal of the American Dietetic Association* 108 (10) (2008): 1716–1731.

33. Tim Byers et al., "American Cancer Society Guidelines on Nutrition and Physical Activity for Cancer Prevention: Reducing the Risk of Cancer with Healthy Food Choices and Physical Activity," *CA: A Cancer Journal for Clinicians* 52, 2 (March/April 2002): 92–119.

34. Ronald M. Krauss et al., "AHA Dietary Guidelines: Revision 2000: A Statement for Healthcare Professionals from the Nutrition Committee of the American Heart Association," *Circulation* 102 (2000): 2284–2299

35. Paul E. Szmitko et al., "Red Wine and Your Heart," *Circulation* 111 (2005): e10-e11.

36. http://www.cdc.gov/alcohol/fact-sheets/binge-drinking. htm

Organic or Not?

1. Michael C. Alavanja et al., "The Agricultural Health Study," *Environmental Health Perspectives* 104, no. 4 (April 1996): 362–369.

2. Crystal Smith-Spangler et al., "Are Organic Foods Safer or Healthier than Conventional Alternatives?" *Annals of Internal Medicine* 157, no. 5 (Sept. 4, 2012): 1–W-4.

3. http://npic.orst.edu/factsheets/ddttech.pdf

4. http://www.fda.gov/Food/GuidanceComplianceRegulatoryInformation/GuidanceDocuments/Biotechnology/ucm096095.htm

5. http://www.ama-assn.org/resources/doc/csaph/a12-csaph2-bioengineeredfoods.pdf

6. http://aaemonline.org/gmopost.html

Part III:
Let's Dive In!

Let's Compare, Shall We?

1. "The Price of a Heart Attack," *The Washington Post* (2009). http://www.washingtonpost.com/wp-dyn/content/graphic/2009/07/26/GR2009072600010.html.

2. "Fats and Oils: AHA Recommendation," *American Heart Association* http://www.heart.org/HEARTORG/GettingHealthy/FatsAndOils/Fats101/Fats-and-Oils-AHA-Recommendation_UCM_316375_Article.jsp.

Supplementation or Not?

1. Maria T. Cerqueira et al., "The Food and Nutrient Intakes of the Tarahumara Indians of Mexico," *The American Journal of Clinical Nutrition* (April 1979): 905–915.

2. Second National Report on Biochemical Indicators of Diet and Nutrition in the U.S. Population, Executive Summary, 2012 CDC National Center for Environmental Health. Available at http://www.cdc.gov/nutritionreport/

3. J. J. Kastlelein et al., "Simvastatin With or Without Ezetimibe in Familial Hypercholesterolemia," *N Engl J Med* 358, no. 14 (April 3, 2008): 1431–1443.

4. Jeanne Lenzer, "Unreported Cholesterol Drug Data Released by Company," *BMJ* (British Medical Journal), 336, no. 7637 (2008): 180–181.

5. http://www.fda.gov/food/ResourcesForYou/Consumers/
    NFLPM/ucm274593.htm#dvs

6. http://ods.od.nih.gov/factsheets/VitaminB6-HealthPro-
    fessional/

7. Charles R. Scriver and J. H. Hutchison, "The Vitamin B6
    Deficiency Syndrome in Human Infancy: Biochemical
    and Clinical Observations," *Pediatrics* 31, no. 2 (February
    1, 1963): 240–250.

8. http://www.nlm.nih.gov/medlineplus/iron.html

9. Peter A. Chyka and Adrianne Y. Butler "Assessment of
    Acute Iron Poisoning by Laboratory and Clinical Obser-
    vations," *The American Journal of Emergency Medicine* 11, 2
    (March 1993): 99–103.

10. http://www.nlm.nih.gov/medlineplus/ency/arti-
    cle/002404.htm

11. Laura Pimentel, "Scurvy: Historical Review and Current
    Diagnostic Approach," *Amer. J. Emergency Medicine* 21,
    no. 4 (2003): 328–330.

12. R. M. Douglas et al., "Vitamin C for Preventing and
    Treating the Common Cold," *Cochrane Database Syst.
    Rev.* (3) (July 18, 2007): CD000980.

13. J. Verrax and P. Buc Calderon, "The Controversial Place of
    Vitamin C in Cancer Treatment," *Biochemical Pharmacol-
    ogy* 76, 12 (December 15, 2008): 1644–1652.

14. L. J. Hoffer et al., "Phase I Clinical Trial of IV Ascorbic
    Acid in Advanced Malignancy," *Annals of Oncology* 19, no.
    11 (2008): 1969–1974.

15. http://www.nlm.nih.gov/medlineplus/ency/article/002404.htm

16. Eric N. Taylor et al., "Dietary Factors and the Risk of Incident Kidney Stones in Men: New Insights After 14 Years of Follow-Up," *Journal of the American Society of Nephrology* 15, no. 12 (2004): 3225–3232.

17. Olivier Traxer et al., "Effect of Ascorbic Acid Consumption on Urinary Stone Risk Factors," *Clinical Urology* 170, 2, Part 1 (August 2003): 397–401.

18. http://ods.od.nih.gov/factsheets/VitaminB12-Quick-Facts/

19. http://www.nlm.nih.gov/medlineplus/ency/article/002400.htm

20. M. Ezzati et al., "Comparative Quantification of Health Risks: Global and Regional Burden of Diseases Attributable to Selected Major Risks," The World Health Organization (2004).

21. Adrianne Bendich and Lillian Langseth, "Safety of Vitamin A," *Am J Clin Nutr* 49, no. 2 (February 1989): 358–371.

22. http://ods.od.nih.gov/factsheets/VitaminE-HealthProfessional/

23. M. J. Stampfer et al., "Vitamin E Consumption and the Risk of Coronary Disease in Women," *N Engl J Med* 328 (1993): 1444–1449.

24. M. G. Traber et al., "Heart Disease and Single-Vitamin Supplementation," *Am J Clin Nutr* 85 (2007): 293S–299S.

25. I. Jialal and S. Devaraj, "Vitamin E Supplementation and Cardiovascular Events in High-Risk Patients," *N Engl J Med* 342 (2000): 154–160.

26. E. Lonn et al., "Effects of Long-Term Vitamin E Supplementation on Cardiovascular Events and Cancer: A Randomized Controlled Trial," *JAMA* 293 (2005): 1338–1347.

27. B. G. Brown and J. Crowley, "Is There Any Hope for Vitamin E?" *JAMA* 293 (2005):1387–1390.

28. I-M Lee et al., "Vitamin E in the Primary Prevention of Cardiovascular Disease and Cancer: The Woman's Health Study: A Randomized, Controlled Trial," *JAMA* 294 (2005): 56–65.

29. H. D. Sesso et al., "Vitamins E and C in the Prevention of Cardiovascular Disease in Men: The Physician's Health Study II Randomized Controlled Trial," *JAMA* 300 (2008): 2123–2133.

30. P. Knekt et al., "Antioxidant Vitamin Intake and Coronary Mortality in a Longitudinal Population Study," *Am. J. Epidemiol* 139 (1994): 1180–1189.

31. Scott M. Lippman et al., "Effect of Selenium and Vitamin E on Risk of Prostate Cancer and Other Cancers," *JAMA* 301, no. 1 (2009): 39–51.

32. R. M. Bostick et al., "Reduced Risk of Colon Cancer with High Intakes of Vitamin E: The Iowa Women's Health Study," *Cancer Res* 15 (1993): 4230–4317.

33. K. Wu, et al., "A Prospective Study on Supplemental Vitamin E Intake and Risk of Colon Cancer in Men and

Women," *Cancer Epidemiol Biomarkers Prev* 11 (2002): 1298–1304.

34. Edgar R. Miller III et al., "Meta-Analysis: High-Dosage Vitamin E Supplementation May Increase All-Cause Mortality," *Annals of Internal Medicine* 142, no. 1 (2005): 37–46.

35. http://www.nlm.nih.gov/medlineplus/ency/article/000354.htm

36. TPA Devasagayam et al., "Free Radicals and Antioxidants in Human Health: Current Status and Future Prospects," *JAPI* 52 (October 2004).

37. Gilbert S. Omenn et al., "Effects of a Combination of Beta Carotene and Vitamin A on Lung Cancer and Cardiovascular Disease," *New England Journal of Medicine* 334 (May 2, 1996): 1150–1155.

38. Yun-Zhong Fang et al., "Free Radicals, Antioxidants, and Nutrition," *Nutrition* 18 (2002): 872–879.

39. Rui Hai Liu, "Health Benefits of Fruit and Vegetables are from Additive and Synergistic Combinations of Phytochemicals," *Am J Clin Nutr* 78 (suppl) (2003): 517S–520S.

40. R. L. Lester and F. L. Crane, "The Natural Occurrence of Coenzyme Q and Related Compounds," *The Journal of Biological Chemistry* 234, no. 8 (1959): 2169–2175.

41. Paul S. Watson et al., "Lack of Effect of Coenzyme Q on Left Ventricular Function in Patients with Congestive Heart Failure," *Journal of the American College of Cardiology* 33 (1999):1549–1552.

42. C. Morisco et al., "Effect of Coenzyme Q10 Therapy in Patients With Congestive Heart Failure: A Long-Term

Multicenter Randomized Study," *The Clinical Investigator* 71, 8 (suppl) (1993): S134–S136

43. Franklin Rosenfeldt et al., "Coenzyme Q Therapy Before Cardiac Surgery Improves Mitochondrial Function and In Vitro Contractility of Myocardial Tissue," *The Journal of Thoracic and Cardiovascular Surgery* 129, no. 1 (2005): 25–32.

44. Romualdo Belardinelli et al., "Coenzyme Q and Exercise Training in Chronic Heart Failure," *European Heart Journal*, 27 (2006): 2675–2681.

45. S. A. Mortensen et. al., "Dose-Related Decrease of Serum Coenzyme Q_{10} During Treatment With HMG-Coa Reductase Inhibitors," *Molecular Aspects of Medicine* 18 (Suppl.) 1 (1997): 137–144.

46. Leo Marcoff and Paul D. Thompson, "The Role of Coenzyme Q in Statin-Induced Myopathy: A Systematic Review," *Journal of the American College of Cardiology* 49, 23 (2007): 2231–2237.

47. Marcia Wyman, et al., "Coenzyme Q: A Therapy for Hypertension and Statin-Induced Myalgia?" *Cleveland Clinic Journal of Medicine* 77, no. 7 (2010): 435–442.

48. V. L. Serebruany et al., "Dietary Coenzyme Q Supplementation Alters Platelet Size and Inhibits Human Vitronectin (CD51/CD61) Receptor Expression," *Journal of Cardiovascular Pharmacology* 29 (1997): 16–22.

49. A.M. Heck et al., "Potential Interactions Between Alternative Therapies and Warfarin," *American Journal of Health-System Pharmacy*, 57, no. 13 (2000): 1221–1227.

50. P. Langsjoen et al., "Treatment of essential hypertension with Coenzyme Q_{10}." *Molecular Aspects of Medicine* 15 (Suppl.), 1 (1994): s265–s272.

51. J. M. Hodgson et al., "Coenzyme Q Improves Blood Pressure and Glycaemic Control: A Controlled Trial in Subjects with Type 2 Diabetes," *European Journal of Clinical Nutrition* 56 (2002): 1137—1142.

Exercise and Sleep

1. T. S. Church et al., "Exercise Without Weight Loss Does Not Reduce C-Reactive Protein: The INFLAME Study," *Med Sci Sports Exerc* 4, no. 4 (2010): 708–716.

2. L. H. Colbert et al., "Physical Activity, Exercise, and Inflammatory Markers in Older Adults: Findings from the Health, Aging, and Body Composition Study," *Journal of the American Geriatrics Society* 52 (2004): 1098–1104.

3. S. P. Whelton et al., "Effect Of Aerobic Exercise on Blood Pressure: A Meta-Analysis of Randomized, Controlled Trials, *Annals of Internal Medicine* 36, no. 7 (2002): 493–503.

4. Robert H. Fagard and Vérnonique A. Cornelisson, "Effect of Exercise on Blood Pressure Control in Hypertensive Patients," *European Journal of Preventive Cardiology* 14, no. 1 (2007): 12–17.

5. Jang-Rak Kim et al., "Effect of Exercise Intensity and Frequency on Lipid Levels in Men with Coronary Heart Disease: Training Level Comparison Trial," *The American Journal of Cardiology* 87, 8 (2001): 942–946.

6. "American Diabetes Association Mission Statement: Standards of Medical Care in Diabetes, 2012," *Diabetes Care* 35, Supplement 1 (January 2012).

7. Jennifer K. Cooney et al., "Benefits of Exercise on Rheumatoid Arthritis," *Journal of Aging Research* 2011, Article ID 681640 (2011).

8. Janet M. Mullington et al., "Cardiovascular, Inflammatory and Metabolic Consequences of Sleep Deprivation," *Prog Cardiovasc Dis.* 51, no. 4 (2009): 294–302.

Part IV:
Strategies for Specific Medical Issues

Prediabetes and Type 2 Diabetes Mellitus

1. http://www.lancet.com/journals/lancet/article/PIIS0140-6736(10)61011-2/fulltext

2. "Diabetes Prevention Program Research Group (2002) Reduction in the Incidence of Type 2 Diabetes with Lifestyle Intervention or Metformin," *The New England Journal of Medicine* 346, no. 6: 393–403.

3. "American Diabetes Association Mission Statement: Standards of Medical Care in Diabetes, 2012," *Diabetes Care*, Vol. 35, Supplement 1, January 2012.

Cardiovascular Disease

1. Donald Lloyd Jones et al., "Heart Disease and Stroke Statistics—2009 Update: A Report from the American Heart Association Statistics Committee and Stroke

Statistics Subcommittee," *Circulation* 119 (2009): 480–486.

2. Kimberly G. Thigpen, "Fighting Obesity through the Built Environment," *Environmental Health Perspectives*, 112, no. 11 (2004): A616–A619.

3. Samuel S. Gidding et al., "Implementing American Heart Association Pediatric and Adult Nutrition Guidelines," *Circulation* 119 (2009): 1161–1175.

Chronic Kidney Disease

1. http://www.kidney.org/kidneydisease/aboutckd.cfm

2. Andrew S. Levey et al., "National Kidney Foundation Practice Guidelines for Chronic Kidney Disease: Evaluation, Classification, and Stratification," *Annals of Internal Medicine* 139 (2003): 137–147.

3. Mary Width and Tonia Reinhard, *The Clinical Dietitian's Essential Pocket Guide* (2009): 257–270.

Celiac Disease

1. Official Recommendations of the American Gastroen-terological Association Institute (2006) AGA Institute Medical Position Statement on the Diagnosis and Management of Celiac Disease.

2. Mary Width and Tonia Reinhard, *The Clinical Dietitian's Essential Pocket Guide*, (2009): 257–270.

3. Jean A. T. Pennington and Judith Spungen, *Food Values of Portions Commonly Used*, 19 ed. (Lippincott Williams and Wilkins, 2010).

Diverticulosis

1. http://digestive.niddk.nih.gov/ddiseases/pubs/diverticu-losis/diverticulosis_508.pdf

2. Mary Width and Tonia Reinhard (2009) *The Clinical Dietitian's Essential Pocket Guide*, pp. 257—270.

Part V:
Become Your Own Scientist

1. Stephen Bent, "Herbal Medicine in the United States: Review of Efficacy, Safety, and Regulation," *J Gen Intern Med* 23 (6) (2008): 854–859.

2. J. L. Nortier et al., "Urothelial Carcinoma Associated with the Use of a Chinese Herb (*Aristolochia fangchi*), *N Engl J Med* 342, (2000): 1686–1692.

3. Stephen Bent, "The Relative Safety of Ephedra Compared with Other Herbal Products," *Ann Intern Med* 138 (2003): 468–471.

4. Paul G. Shekelle et al., "Efficacy and Safety of Ephedra and Ephedrine for Weight Loss and Athletic Performance: A Meta-Analysis," *JAMA* 289, (12) (March 26, 2003): 1537–1545.

What Is Good Science?

1. Esteban Walker et al., "Meta-analysis: Its Strengths and Limitations," *Cleveland Clinic Journal of Medicine* 75, no. 6 (2008): 431–439.

2. E. H. Turner, et al., "Selective Publication of Antidepressant Trials and its Influence on Apparent Efficacy," *N Engl J Med* 358 (2008): 252–260.

The Dietary Supplement Industry: Does the Government Protect You?

1. 21 U.S.C. § 342—Adulterated Food. http://www.law.cornell.edu/U.S.code/text/21/342

2. 21 U.S.C. § 351—Adulterated Drugs and Devices. http://www.law.cornell.edu/U.S.code/text/21/351

3. "How Drugs Are Developed And Approved," FDA.gov. April 2010. U.S. Food and Drug Administration. October 31, 2012. http://www.fda.gov/drugs/developmentapprovalprocess/howdrugsaredevelopedandapproved/default.htm

4. Charles Adams and Van Brantner, "New Drug Development: Estimating Entry From Human Clinical Trials," Bureau of Economics, Federal Trade Commission. July 7, 2003. http://www.ftc.gov/be/workpapers/wp262.pdf

5. Id.

6. Jane Henney, "Implementation of The Dietary Supplement Health And Education Act (DSHEA) of 1994." FDA.gov. March 25, 1999. U.S. Food and Drug Administration. October 20, 2012. http://www.fda.gov/NewsEvents/Testimony/ucm115082.htm

7. Id.

8. "Utah Nutritional Products Industry Profile." EDCUtah.org. 2009. Economic Development Corporation Of Utah.

October 20, 2012. http://www.edcutah.org/files/Utah_Nutritional_Products_Industry_Profile_09.pdf

9. Carolyn McClanahan, "How Much Should We Spend On Health Care? The Big Picture," Forbes.com. November 28, 2011. Forbes. http://www.forbes.com/sites/carolynmcclanahan/2011/1½8/how-much-should-we-spend-on-health-care-the-big-picture/

10. Dietary Supplement Health And Education Act of 1994, 21 U.S.C 301, (1994)

11. Eric Lipton, "Support Is Mutual for Senator and Utah Industry,"NYTimes.com.June20,2011.*TheNewYorkTimes.* October 20, 2012. http://www.nytimes.com/2011/06/21/U.S./politics/21hatch.html?pagewanted=all

12. 21 C.F.R. § 101.72.

13. "Guidance for Industry: Structure/Function Claims, Small Entity Compliance Guide," FDA.gov. January 9, 2002. U.S. Food and Drug Administration. November 13, 2012. http://www.fda.gov/Food/GuidanceComplianceRegulatoryInformation/GuidanceDocuments/DietarySupplements/ucm103340.htm

14. Id.

15. "Dangerous Supplements: What Your Don't Know About These 12 Ingredients Could Hurt You." Consumerreports.org. September 2010. Consumer Reports. October 20, 2012. http://www.consumerreports.org/cro/2012/05/dangerous-supplements/index.htm

16. Id.

17. Id.

18. "Recalls, Market Withdrawals, & Safety Alerts Search." FDA.gov. U.S. Food and Drug Administration. October 30, 2012. http://www.fda.gov/Safety/Recalls/default.htm

19. "Uva Ursi." UMM.edu. 2011. University of Maryland Medical Center. November 6, 2012. www.umm.edu/altmed/articles/uva-ursi-000278.htm

20. "Kava Kava." UMM.edu. 2011. University of Maryland Medical Center. November 6, 2012. http://www.umm.edu/altmed/articles/kava-kava-000259.htm

21. "Dangerous Supplements: What Your Don't Know About These 12 Ingredients Could Hurt You." Consumerreports.org. September 2010. Consumer Reports. October 20, 2012. http://www.consumerreports.org/cro/2012/05/dangerous-supplements/index.htm

22. "Colloidal Silver." Nccam.nih.gov. February 2012. National Center for Complementary and Alternative Medicine at the National Institutes of Health. November 6, 2012. http://nccam.nih.gov/health/silver

23. Id.

24. Miranda Hitti, "Colloidal Silver: FAQ," September 2008. Webmd.com. November 6, 2012. http://www.webmd.com/news/20080905/colloidal-silver-faq

25. "Dietary Supplements: An Advertising Guide for Industry," FTC.gov, April 2001, Federal Trade Commission, Bureau of Consumer Protection. October 20, 2012. http://business.ftc.gov/documents/bus09-dietary-supplements-advertising-guide-industry

26. Id.

INDEX

· ·

E   F

T